THE NHS AND IDEOLOGICAL CONFLICT

The NHS and Ideological Conflict

PAUL HIGGS

Avebury

Aldershot · Brookfield USA · Hong Kong · Singapore · Sydney

Published by
Avebury
Ashgate Publishing Limited
Gower House
Croft Road
Aldershot
Hants GU11 3HR
England

Ashgate Publishing Company
Old Post Road
Brookfield
Vermont 05036
USA

A CIP catalogue record for this book is available from the British Library

ISBN 1 85628 346 1

Printed and Bound in Great Britain by
Athenaeum Press Ltd., Newcastle upon Tyne.

Contents

Acknowledgements

I would like to thank my supervisor Professor Peter Taylor-Gooby for his help and guidance while I undertook the study that this book is based upon. I would also like to thank Professor Peter Millard for allowing me the time to turn the study into this book. Many friends helped at different stages in the completion of both of these tasks, sometimes by offering encouragement. Special thanks, however, must go to Rachel Reed who proof read much of this book and offered invaluable criticism on style, grammar and comprehension. The research was undertaken as a part of a PhD at the University of Kent at Canterbury and was supported by an ESRC studentship.

1 The theory and practice of counter-hegemonic struggle

It is the argument of this book that the labour movement's response to privatisation in the mid-1980s displayed a new approach towards politics that gained ascendancy among sections of the Labour Party and of the left. In many ways it prepared the ground for the policy orientations contained within Labour's "Policy Review" of the late 1980s. It was a strategy that started from a belief in the need to fight political struggles at the level of "values" and emphasised the importance of the construction of an ideological counter- offensive to "Thatcherism".

The privatisation of parts of the NHS was important to this counter-offensive because it allowed Labour and the left to stress the "collective" values of the NHS against the "individualistic" ones of privatisation. Although the Labour party has never been explicitly left-wing or Marxist, it is interesting to note that many of the ideas underlying this strategy have their origin in theoretical developments within contemporary neo-Marxism, which in turn regarded it as alternative to theories based on "economism" or uninspiring "Labourism".

The significance of industrial action by NHS ancillary workers against privatisation was that strikes could be a focus for such an ideological campaign, in that they were a practical reminder of the value conflict that exists between collectivism and individualism. This in turn could be translated into political capital for the Labour Party (for this strategy meant nothing if it was not aimed at electoral power). However, when

1

NHS workers took industrial action against privatisation and especially when they went on indefinite strike, they had either to compromise their ability to win the strike or they had to ditch their emphasis on winning over public opinion. This followed from the nature of industrial action in a public service such as a hospital where the "product" affected was the public and its health care needs. The tension between these two strategies is such that in studying examples of where they were in collision we can get a fuller picture of the effectiveness of giving priority to conflict at the level of public opinion. In turn, the results of the contradiction between these two forms of opposition to privatisation can also illuminate the theory of ideology and the question of political consciousness. Before we can do that we must look at the origins of this counter-hegemonic strategy.

The welfare state and the NHS

Much was written about the dominance of "New Right" ideas during the 1980s. Writers such as Hall (1983) described the emergence of authoritarian and anti-collectivist sentiment among large sections of the population during the 1970s. Golding and Middleton (1982) wrote about the anti-welfare backlash. Everywhere there was talk of the "crisis of the welfare state". It was argued that the institutions of the Beveridgian welfare state had lost popular support and that there had been a growth of self-interested individualism. The causes for this state of affairs was attributed to many factors, not least the failure of the welfare state to solve the problems that it was supposed to eradicate.

This brought to the forefront of discussion the whole question of what the welfare state stood for and it is within this discussion that the ideological importance of the welfare state occurs. For while the terms of academic debate are centred on the validity of assumptions, intentions, inputs, and ethical outcomes of the social services (see Rawls (1972), Nozick (1974), and Weale (1986)), the debate as it occurred at an everyday level was (and is) essentially political in composition. It derives its importance from the articulation of the differing forms in which basic human needs are met. As George and Wilding point out:

> If it is to flourish, any economic system both requires and generates a particular value system. Capitalism is no exception. It depends on and fosters the development of an ethic of self-help, freedom, individualism, competition and achievement - the classical liberal values.

2

Such a value system, which is required for the successful operation of a capitalist economy, is in clear opposition to the values needed to underpin a successful public welfare system. If such a system is to flourish, the stress on the virtue of self-help must be replaced by the stress on the need to help others. Individualism must be replaced by a concern for the community at large; competition by co-operation; achievement must be defined in social and communal rather than in individual terms - values that are socialist rather than liberal. The economic system and the welfare system, therefore, require and depend on quite different value systems. Conflict between economic and social purposes and between liberal and social values is therefore inherent in capitalist society.

(George and Wilding, 1976, p118)

Moreover, as they go on to argue, there has always existed a conflict between these two approaches in the field of social policy. There has been a continual assertion and reassertion of individual freedom over collective responsibility. This varies from the "right" of doctors to continue to practice private medicine in the NHS, to the insurance principle that underlies the majority of social security responsibilities. It is a conflict in which the differing interpretations of equality are of paramount importance. Is it the equality of equal opportunity to compete for scarce resources in an unequal world; or is it the equality of providing everybody with what they need? This is made explicit by those in favour of the welfare state:

One fundamental historical reason for the adoption of this principle (universalism) was the aim of making services available and accessible to the whole population in such ways as would not involve users in any humiliating loss of status, dignity or self respect. There should be no sense of inferiority, pauperism, shame or stigma in the use of a publicly provided service; no attribution that one was being or becoming a "public" burden. Hence the emphasis on the social rights of all citizens to use or not to use as responsible citizens the services made available by the community, which the private market and the family were unable or unwilling to provide universally.

(Titmuss, 1969, p129)

While this conflict of values is seldom admitted in public by those trying to bring market forces into play, it is some times alluded to by them in private. As Jewkes and Jewkes argued in 1980 when advocating making voluntary health insurance premiums deductible from taxable income:

> ...since we all value most that which we pay for, it would help sweep away, after 32 years, the most bizarre socialist dream that has ever bedevilled our people... that the state can provide all and every medical service and medicament... without discouraging economy, creating shortages, and debasing quality.
> (Jewkes and Jewkes, 1980, quoted in Forsyth, 1982,p67)

In Britain, out of all the institutions of the welfare state, it is the NHS that most clearly illustrates this ideological divide. This is because of its emphasis on the equality of treatment regardless of social status or ability to pay. In establishing this principle the NHS went beyond the rationality of the market and moved into the sphere of social production. That is production for need and not for profit.

The growth of individualism as represented by the laissez- faire attitude of the Thatcher governments is a negation of the concept of collective provision. The NHS, because of its association with helping those not in a position, through no fault of their own, to help themselves, is seen as a symbol of an entirely different approach to the concerns of society. And what is even more important is the fact that the NHS is immensely popular because of this principle. Jewkes and Jewkes complained of "the almost pathological obsession on the part of the British public, in the face of all fact and logic, with the indestructible virtues of a comprehensive and free NHS". They conclude "reform will call for patience, step-by-step progress and the use of the thin end of the wedge". Privatisation is such a "thin end of a wedge".

So far, I have outlined the potential for an ideological conflict over the provision of state welfare. But it is the issue of privatisation that brings such a conflict out into the open. Why is this? It could be argued that this contradiction might apply to such principles as universal provision as against individual insurance in the supply of medical cover, but that its relevance to the letting out of private contracts to clean hospitals is another matter altogether. Certainly, there is an amount of truth in this. At two of the hospitals where interviews were conducted and where industrial action against the tender had occurred, private contractors already had had a foothold in the running of cleaning services long before the current controversy had begun. In one case the private contract had been in place since the 1960s. However, privatisation is more than just a re-adjustment of working practices. Instead it involves the articulation of fundamentally different principles and priorities. This can be seen, not only in terms of the Jewkes's "thin wedge", but also

4

through the undeniably "ideological" form that the disputes took; in the views of the ancillary workers themselves and in the nature of the publicity that resulted. The question of privatisation and the conflict of social values is one that is inextricably linked to the whole competitive tendering process.

This book will therefore be concerned with looking at the ways in which the ancillary workers themselves viewed the processes of privatisation and to what extent they saw a conflict of values. This will concentrate not only on what they said, but also the way in which they said it, and the degree to which they constructed a coherent view of their predicament. This will be important because, any strategy so convinced of the political importance of values should be able to regard this group as establishing its bedrock support given privatised workers' pragmatic interest in its success.

Ideology and public sector workers

One of the most important reasons why the strategy of ideological struggle was adopted in the fight against privatisation is to do with the social nature of the work that ancillary workers do. However, it is a long distance between acknowledging this fact and seeing the need to develop a strategy geared to winning over public opinion. The evolution of this process has a complicated history, much of it to do with the decline in confidence that many rank-and-file trade unionists experienced with their own ability to affect change. But what is also of importance has been the development of theories on the left which have seen public sector workers occupying special positions in the mode of production - positions that gave them different abilities (and different responsibilities) to those of the traditional working class. While none of these theories were so explicit as to claim that industrial struggle needed to be replaced by ideological struggle, their work as a whole did lead in this direction. In what follows I will try to show how this movement in ideas has occurred.

The starting point for most writers is the premise that public sector workers do not have a completely symmetrical correspondence with those working in the private sector insofar as the nature of their work is concerned. This in turn leads to the proposition that, in fact, public employees have different ideological pressures operating on them; pressures that lead intrinsically to the creation of counter-hegemonic positions. In other words, they are likely to develop ideas that oppose the legitimacy of capitalist market principles in and through their work.

The reason that this group is subject to the influence of these counter-hegemonic positions is a result of the functions that this group of workers perform for society as a whole. The fact that much public sector employment is not geared directly to the creation of profits, but to the servicing of need, lessens the impact of market derived ideology. As Therborn writes: "The concerns of reproductive workers and employees have nothing directly to do with the accumulation of capital, they are geared to human relations, rather than commodities" (Therborn, 1984, p34).

Public employees are placed in a situation where the abstract questions of political principle become practical and relevant, and where the values of the welfare state become their values. Many writers go further and argue that those working in the "public services" are in fact decommodified because they produce no profit and can therefore break out of the ideological straight-jacket of commodity fetishism - thus realising that economic questions are simultaneously political ones.

> Class struggle over the nature and size of state goods and services cannot be strictly economistic. This is because most state workers such as teachers, health workers, social workers, are struggling over conditions of work and more services which directly affect their object of production - that is, other people, for example, students pensioners and the sick. Every attack upon the definition and organisation of education, health transport, etc., is a struggle over social relations in a way that narrow wage demands in private factories are not.
> (Frankel, 1976, pp60-61)

As a result, some (such as Frankel above) can argue that these workers represent the vanguard of modern political movements in that their struggles automatically take on a political dimension. Therborn writing about the demise of the industrial proletariat makes this claim; "However, the new stage of advanced capitalism has also generated new forces of the Left, above all in the public sector unions and the sphere of *socialized reproduction*" (Therborn, 1984, p34, emphasis in original). He goes on to extend this, and make a significant point about the role of ideology in creating the new found importance of this group:

> These reproductive workers and employees are not locked into a direct and immediate conflict with capital, like the proletariat in the classical sense. On the other hand they play a major role in the new dimension of class struggle, external to, but dependent upon the capital-wage-labour nexus - which differs from commerce or patriarchal family agriculture in that it tends at least partially to pull

the rug of mass support from under the feet of capital.
(Therborn, 1984, p35)

For some thinkers, ideology becomes an important part of the newly discovered social weight of the public sector employee. How does this operate?   One good example, albeit from the more professionally orientated part of the public sector, was provided by a number of self-proclaimed radicals operating in the area of state social work (Statham (1978) Leonard (1981), and Jones (1983)). For these writers, social work was not just a job, but very much a political activity. For them, the very fact that the social worker deals with human relations means that he or she is faced with a political choice every time they become involved in helping one of their clients.

Consequently, the question arises, do they lay the blame for the situations they are dealing with on the individuals concerned, or do they treat them as victims of an economic and political system that can only function by producing the circumstances that lead to their problems. Even in resolving this dilemma, they are faced with another one. Do they, if they see the problem as lying in the nature of society, then try to influence their clients into taking action against the social and political forms that the welfare state generates, and therefore attempt to take them over for their own use? Because of this, Statham (1978) sees the task of "left radicalism" as being to challenge the basis of an institution, its ideology, and in the long run work for a new society. Similarly Leonard (1981) sees the primary objective of "oppositional practice" as making "some contribution of transforming a private experience of poverty and exploitation into an expression of class consciousness" (Leonard, 1981, p92).

No matter what term is used to describe the nature of the activity (left radicalism, oppositional practice etc.) there is a consensus, at least on the left, that social work can play a directly political role in educating people as to the oppressive nature of society. In this way, the political dimension of the job is as important as the economic power that social workers as waged employees possess, if not more so.

It could be argued with a certain amount of validity, that social work is an anomaly in that it is unlike most other jobs in the public sector. It has an exceptional relationship with the people it serves in that it only sees them when they come to grief at the hands of the system. While this may be true, it at the same time misses the point. All jobs in the social reproduction sector, to a greater or lesser degree, depend on the counter-hegemonic dimension to their jobs. The form that this takes though may differ considerably . It is one thing to be able to change ideas, but it is

7

equally, if not more, important to be perceived as being necessary to the community as a whole. And it is necessary to be aware of this other dimension in any discussion of this sector. Therefore, while teachers may be in a position to develop alternatives to the capitalist instrumentality of the examinations system, in the end, it is to public sympathy and popular support that they turn in attempting to achieve their ends. Again, it could be argued that these conditions apply only to the professionalised white-collar end of the spectrum of the public services. Again, there is some truth, but crucially when refuse services, direct works organisations and other manual public sector workers have been affected by government and other action, they too have appealed to the public on ideological grounds. Obviously, there may be an element of pragmatic self-interest in operation here, but, the very fact that such appeals are made, and seem in many cases, to be the only form of action contemplated does suggest the domination of the ideological dimension.

If the above is true, then the impact of struggles in the welfare state will be more important than the impact of economic / political struggles elsewhere. It will also mean the adoption of different forms of organisation from those traditionally used by the labour movement. An influential document produced by the London Edinburgh Weekend Return Group (1979), a group of socialist intellectuals involved in the public sector, argued, in a path breaking fashion that the defence and extension of the welfare state necessitated what they described as as "material counter organisation". In this, the role of consumers as users of public services was crucial. Partly this approach is pre-figurative in that it attempted to challenge "the traditional boundaries between clients and workers and the non-class categories" by attempting to use "ways of relating to each other which are anti-capitalist and at the same time, in a partial and temporary way, also socialist and feminist" (LEWERG, 1979, p50). However what is more important is their attitude to industrial struggle in the public sector. Here the negative side of the public sectors ideological importance is demonstrated. Not only can they pre-figure different forms of social organisation but also, they can hinder it through their own activity. Drawing on the effects of the public sector wage strikes of 1978-79 they write:

> The leadership of the public sector unions reasoned that pressure put on the people by the interruption of public services becomes, indirectly, pressure put on the state, which will then accede to union demands. But in this way the weakest, already suffering from the mean level of state services, doubly suffer from their withdrawal. Even this perverse strategy is not available to certain groups of state

8

workers, who do not have a ready "public" to use as their weapon: research workers, for instance, and community workers.

The impact of the winter strikes on the state and capital was difficult to assess. But many ordinary people, not known for their right wing views, commented that they were hurting ordinary people more than the government. It became clear that, in future periods of industrial action, more imaginative forms of action would have to be developed.

It is not even as if strikes in the public sector have been shown to be particularly successful in their own terms. We cannot pretend that withdrawing labour has the same effect on the state as on private capital. Precisely because it hurts working class people more than the state, such action does not impose very effective sanctions on the state. Taking the private sector as a model is not appropriate.

(LEWERG, 1979, p54)

The result, given its emphasis on symbolic action and tokenistic protest, is an advocacy of what be described as "community politics". This can be seen from the strategies that they emphasise: autonomous struggles; overcoming individualisation; rejecting misleading categories; defining ourselves in class terms; defining our problem our way; stepping outside[1]. the brief; refusing official procedure; rejecting managerial priorities; etc

It could be argued that there is everything to be achieved in politicising conflicts of interest, what has occurred with the LEWERG position is the almost complete replacement of realistic forms of struggle (i.e. traditional "economism") with a form of political consciousness raising which, as I will argue later, is completely inappropriate. If this was the way that the strategy of using ideological struggle as an alternative to industrial action has developed at a theoretical level, it is not true that these thinkers were responsible for its utilisation and consequences. The people who implemented it in the trade union hierarchy were shifting in this direction anyway. The loss of electoral power by Labour in 1979 was seen as a result of the previous years public sector strikes and was therefore the fault of the big public service unions. Undoubtably though, this development which has been dressed up in theoretical terms as "non-reductionist", "anti-economist" and other adjectives of the "New Left", has provided a handy vantage point for the "new realism" of sections of the trade union left.

It is also true to say that nowhere was it being used with more determination than in the anti-privatisation struggles of NHS ancillaries.

9

Here, as the evidence I will provide shows, this was the dominant approach - belying claims to the opposite and even on occasions intentions to the opposite. A candid example of the adoption of the approach is provided in a speech by the national education officer of NUPE on the ambulance workers pay claim:

> Our members haven't got a great deal of muscle, if our members go on strike then people die - and our members won't kill people... All this nonsense about industrial muscle and the power of the trade union movement is just so much rhetoric that we believe. Trade Unionism has no intrinsic power, it might have a bit of bargaining power. But in terms of the sort of power we are talking about it never existed and never will exist in an economy where the employer has the power. The employer says yes or no, I don't have the power to say yes or no to a wage deal. The employer has all the power in the end of the day and workers find themselves in the position workers find themselves today . Their power, where it exists, is to influence people and to influence ideas, and to try and capture masses of people for new ideas and new ways of going about business.

This perspective has as its logical extension the building of alliances between those groups working in the public services and the various outside bodies that together go to make up the "public". The strategy has been at the heart of the campaigns waged by the Royal College of Nursing and the Teaching unions (see Travis, 1987) and is seen as the ideal for struggles in the NHS (see Moor, 1987). Indeed the major NHS disputes of 1989 that prompted Mrs Thatcher's "NHS Review"made a virtue of this strategy.

As has been pointed out, using it entails a down playing of industrial struggle and an emphasis on alternative plans and cross class community involvement. Iliffe (1983) illustrates this tendency of seeing industrial struggle as of secondary importance when he writes: "Militancy, and the widespread support for defence campaigns, depended on the strength of the alternative proposals, and not the other way around" (Iliffe, 1983, p122).

Consequently, this study will be concerned with how, both union officials and rank-and-file members saw the issue of privatisation and how they linked it to wider political issues. It will also be concerned to judge the effects of the strategy of ideological struggle.

Developments in Marxist theory and the status of ideology

In much the same way that the trade union strategy outlined above is underpinned by theoretical arguments concerning the nature of public sector employment, so these positions in turn can be underpinned by recent departures in the fields of ideology and discourse theory. It is difficult to say which came first; the move away from "economism" in the public sector by groups such as LEWERG or, at the more abstract level, the disillusionment of various thinkers with class analysis. However, what can be said is that they have both mutually reinforced one another, each providing justifications for the others existence.

What this means in terms of this research, is that discussion of the effects of treating NHS privatisation as essentially an ideological struggle has a direct bearing on the wider questions of the status of ideology in Marxist theory and on the nature of political consciousness itself.

The theoretical developments that have played such a major part in strengthening the position of the proponents of ideological struggle in the labour movement have, unsuprisingly, their roots in theoretical traditions that have always stressed the importance of communication and ideas; namely linguistics and cultural studies. The influence of these approaches has also been compounded by the crisis of Marxist theory that has occurred since the demise of the "Cultural Revolution" in China in the mid-1970s[2].

In this way, traditional Marxist approaches to political and analytical questions were abandoned in favour of the "relative autonomy of the superstructures" approach, this was accompanied by an acceptance of the indeterminacy of various forms of oppression by the economy (the coupling of capitalism as a mode of production with Patriarchy theory etc.), and in the final instance, by the rejection of the economy as even determinant.

While it is important to note that not all thinkers re-examining Marxist arguments in this way have reached the same conclusions, what it is true to say is that most of them have been influenced, in one way or another, by these views and that as a natural consequence the question of winning hegemony becomes paramount. Once the primacy of the economic has been challenged in theory it is only a short step to the down playing of the importance of class. Poulantzas in his "Classes in Contemporary Capitalism" (1975) started this particular ball rolling by arguing that ideological factors have a crucial place in locating individuals into classes; especially given the "unproductive" nature of most public sector workers. In this way Poulantzas presents an analysis of class in which relations of exploitation can be secondary factors to those of ideology. The

11

importance of this position, according to Wood (1986), is that if ideology plays such a considerable role in the constitution of class; and if state workers are really members of the "New Petty Bourgeoisie" linked to the "productive" working class only through ideology, then the role of socialist politics is to build alliances between these various groups by attempting to represent all of their interests, and not just those of the traditional working class.

Obviously, this position is linked to that of his well known discription of the state as "the condensation of class interests", where the basic indeterminacy of the capitalist state ensures that a purely constitutional struggle for state power can occur through the medium of winning hegemony.

While Poulantzas at least sees himself as operating within the Marxist tradition, others who have been influenced by him and by the work of Louis Althusser have moved to a point where, in their writings, classes have no economic basis. The most important of these is Paul Hirst who argues that because material interests cannot exist independently of their constitution by ideology and politics, there therefore cannot be any non-discursive material interests. He bases this position on a thorough going critique of the notion of relative autonomy:

> ...the notion of relative *autonomy* is untenable. Once any degree of autonomous action is accorded to political forces as a means of representation vis-a-vis classes of economic agents, then there is no necessary correspondence between the forces that appear in the political (and what they "represent") and economic classes. It is not simply a question of discrepancy (the political means "represent" the class more or less accurately) but of necessary non-correspondence. One cannot, despite Lenin, "read back" - measuring the political forces against what they are supposed to represent. That is to conceive the represented as external to, as the autonomously existent measure of, its means of representation. Classes do not have given "interests", apparent independently of definite parties, ideologies, etc., and against which these parties, ideologies, etc.,can be measured. What the means of representation "represent" does not exist outside the process of representation.
>
> (Hirst, 1977, pp130-131)

What this points to, and the point certainly isn't missed by later thinkers, is that "politics - and socialist politics in particular - cannot be grounded in the material interests of any class, but must be discursively constructed by autonomous ideological and political means out of "negotiable" social identities" (Wood, 1986, p83). Thus the terrain of ideological struggle and hegemony becomes paramount.

> How can it be maintained that economic agents can have interests defined at the economic level which would be represented at a posteriori at the political and ideological levels? In fact, since it is ideology and through politics that interests are defined, that amounts to stating that interests can exist prior to the discourse in which they are formulated and articulated.
>
> (Mouffe, 1983, p21)

As I have been trying to point out, there are strong similarities between what occured in terms of trade union strategy and these innovations in theory. These similarities, based on a tendency to dismiss the existence of class (or at least to minimise its importance in contemporary events), combined with a prioritising of the question of ideology and discourse, do not mean that there is a definite link between the two. Indeed, it would be hard to imagine the average trade union General Secretary curling up in bed with a work by Paul Hirst or Nicos Poulantzas. However, in the wake of the two (now four) Conservative General Election victories of the last decade and a half, significant numbers of intellectuals have turned to these ideas for guidance[3].

They may have rejected much of what has been written, but the idea that filtered down and became accepted wisdom was that the victory of the Conservatives was essentially an ideological one and needed to be combated accordingly. To make this end feasible new theories (or re-worked old ones) have been developed. They put an emphasis on ideology, alliance building and the re-interpretation of history. Among those attempting to redefine politics in this way are such influential thinkers as Ernesto Laclau, Chantal Mouffe, Eric Hobsbawm, Gareth Stedman-Jones, Barry Hindess, Gavin Kitching and to a lesser extent Stuart Hall. Described variously as the "New Revisionists" (Miliband, 1985) or the "New True Socialists" (NTS)(Wood, 1986), what they share in common is an attempt to redefine the nature of socialist politics by broadening its appeal.

This current is best exemplified by the work of Laclau and Mouffe in their "Hegemony and Socialist Strategy" (1985) where they attempt to combine the Gramscian notion of Hegemony with the benefits of post-structuralism. Following on from Hirst, they argue that as economic interests can only be understood though discourse, political interests too, are created in this realm. Consequently, ideology is the principle level of explanation in society. From this they draw the logical conclusion that the only way to effect social change is to create a universalising discourse that can appeal to all the variously created "subjects" in terms of their own determinations. All the different oppressed and discriminated groups (Women, Black people, Gays and Lesbians, the Handicapped etc.) can retain their own "relative autonomy" of action whilst being a component part of a wider movement. As a result, the problem for socialists of relating to non-class movements is removed. By adopting this strategy, it is no longer necessary to subordinate them to the "wider struggle"; they have now an equal role.

For Laclau and Mouffe this universalising discourse is the concept of democracy. It is by appealing to people on the basis of a new "radical democracy" that sectional interests can be overcome. Central to this proposition is the fact that individuals are not created with a unitary determination, they do in fact have multiple locations and influences:

> Each individual as participant in a series of different social relations is therefore the locus of a plurality of determinations to which correspond subjective positions constructed through discourses and practices with their corresponding "interests". Among those positionalities there is no apriori reason to attribute a special privilege to class, as the articulation principle of subjectivity and determinant of political consciousness. Which positionality will play that role will depend on the discursive practices in which an individual is inserted, and the type of antagonism and of subjectivity they construct.
> (Laclau and Mouffe, 1982, p108)

These notions have been utilised by Hall (1987) and by Lash and Urry (1987) in both "Marxism Today" and "New Socialist" to argue for the abandonment of any appeal to class in politics. Hall argues that "the left, in its organised, labourist form, does not seem to have the slightest conception of what putting together a new historical project entails. It does not understand the necessarily contradictory nature of human subjects, of social identities". Moreover, it does not concentrate on creating "the profound cultural transformation required to *remake* the English" that represents socialism today (Hall, 1987, p21). In all of this "class struggle" is always surrounded by inverted commas. Similarly, Lash and Urry, in the theoretical magazine of the Labour Party itself, argue that not only are white workers and male trade unionists as much "main enemies" as the capitalist crisis and the state bureaucracies themselves, but, that the existence of the labour movement may be an obstacle to the full flowering of pluralistic points of opposition. They conclude the article by praising the virtues of "radical individualism" and see it as the only valid response to a 'disorganised capitalism" where class has no political efficacy. While all of this may be an overstated position, it does represent the trend of thinking.

This exists as a theoretical counterpart to the practical politics of the unions and of the Labour Party during this period (and Later). The appeals to "consensus" and to "capturing the middle ground" are in this light, part of thorough going strategy exemplified by the success of Ken Livingstone's "Save the GLC" campaign. The crucial factor for the campaign's advocates was its effectiveness in mobilising elements traditionally outside the ambit of left-wing politics. Little is said of its failure, however, to actually save the GLC or about the lack of public response to its eventual dismantlement.

The culmination of this theoretical movement can be seen in the promotion of the "New Times" theories championed by the Communist Party in the late 1980s. Drawing extensively on much of the work elaborated above but buttressed by the idea of "post-fordism" (ie the end of an industrial capitalism based on mass production) the proponents of "New Times" promote a political strategy aimed at a non-class reductionist socialism. At its heart lies the idea of hegemonic alliance building linking the political left with the new social movements.

A sense of common purpose between these different social groups will only be developed if they can orientate themselves around a vision of progress which they can share: a common ideological home for progressive politics. New values and visions of progress are emerging from the new times which are strikingly different from Thatcherism's ideology of regressive modernisation. These ideas are both are the product of both the modernisation of established movements such as the trade unions, and the new movements which are emerging such as the green movement. Progressive politics must realign itself around an ideology informed by the progressive values of new times.
(Communist Party, 1989, p13)

Stuart Hall (1989) writing on the importance of this re-orientation cites the issues surrounding health and the NHS as an opportunity to "construct a majoritarian politics of the left". This would be partly done by means of "ideological contestation" of the values on which Thatcherism was built, but also by the construction of a majority based on heterogeneous social interests. This would mean that health and health issues would be radically transformed.

If [the left] knew how to articulate these new forces within the great

15

levelling experience of illness, which hits every one sooner or later irrespective of wealth or class or sexual preference, it would soon discover that society, looked at in a more diversified way, is not at all passive about new needs in the field of health and medical care.
(Hall, 1989, p282)

In this way the ideas of "Marxism Today" take us back to the issues of the struggle over health care. The criticism that such an approach is hardly radical in any meaningful sense is obvious. Be this as it may, for all its faults the new revisionism does make a case that needs answering. It would be easy to dismiss their ideas as theoretical cover for a shift to the right amongst groups of previously euro- communist leaning intellectuals; and certainly there is a grain of truth in this argument. Indeed, the attempts at resurrecting the disastrous Popular Front strategy of Stalin and Dimitriov (which is almost identical in outcome to the present arguments) came from journals such as Marxism Today who have been hawking it in various forms since the nineteen thirties, and for whom there has always been a lot of scope for "progressive alliances". However, as pointed out earlier, to dismiss these ideas purely for this reason would be a mistake because of the influence of this school of thought. Therefore, in criticising these approaches what I intend to show is how many of the ideas of left-wing political strategy, which seem value-free, have in fact serious political consequences. In particular, the notion that appeal to general principles is a higher form of politics than mere "economism" and will therefore produce better results.

The central theme of this work will be that it is impossible to win cultural hegemony for the left if this struggle is only waged at an ideological level. Instead, it will argue that political consciousness cannot be cut off so completely from the material world. To do so is not only to end up in an idealist dead-end, but it is also to be incapable of understanding the reality of peoples' opinions and how these may motivate particular conclusions. As an alternative, I will be arguing for a conception of ideology which is much closer to that of the mainstream Marxist tradition. One which is based on the premise that it is the practical activities of human individuals that are crucial in the development of their opinions; and that these human activities simultaneously produce an understanding of the social world which also has the potential for a rejection of capitalism's priorities on the basis of the different interests of the working class from their rulers.

The successful development of counter-hegemonic opinions depends on the existence of practical activities that reinforce those ideas. For Marxists these activities are those where class conflict is inherent and

16

this will be especially true of strikes.

This is because of the feeling of power that develops out of strike activity among workers is one which strengthens the impact and hold of counter-hegemonic ideas by making practical what is latent in their day to day experiences. From this basis there is the potential for different understandings of the nature of the whole of society.

This makes this research doubly pertinent. Not only does it describe a particular strategy being pursued by the leaders of the labour movement, it also describes how this actually works against the development of the consciousness that they are so eager to attain in their members. This result is reached through the union leaderships limiting the practical activity of workers willing to take industrial action against privatisation. In other words, in dismissing strike action as an ineffective strategy. In this way I shall be arguing for a conception of ideology which is linked to the practical self-activity of human individuals as class subjects and which, accordingly, understands the fluidity and contradictory nature of peoples' thought.

Before we can go on to discuss this, however, we must first understand the pressures that bring about privatisation. The next chapter discusses explanations of the growth of state welfare expenditure and the arguments for its curbing which in turn lead to strategies of privatisation.

Notes

1. These ideas in differing forms are also developed by writers such as Cockburn (1977), Johnson (1978), Iliffe (1983), Boddy and Fudge (1984), and Hain (1985). What they are all concerned with is overcoming "economism" and replacing it with a "political" or "new" trade unionism. Drawing together these arguments, Hain suggests that by developing alternatives to workplace based industrial struggle, and by involving consumers and the new social movements in a broader class struggle alliance, it is possible to move forward. He writes: "What this strategy of building wider alliances offers is not a guarantee of success, but a better prospect of mobilizing broader support and thereby transforming the *political conditions* surrounding attacks on working class interests" (Hain, 1985. p312).

2. For fuller account of this process see Callinicos (1983), Anderson (1983), Wood (1986); for an account of the collapse of Maoism on organised left politics see Harman (1979).

3. Significantly, an article written by in the Guardian to commemorate the 50th anniversary of Antonio Gramsci's death has the following to say about the relevancy of Gramsci's notion of hegemony: "The lessons for the Left were clear. The Labour movement should take stock of the enormity of its ideological and political defeat by the new Thatcherite consensus, and knuckle under to a slow, painful process of constructing its own hegemonic package.Bennite or Scargillite "adventurism" was out. Geldof's Band Aid was the kind of politics that could sweep the land. All this chimed in neatly with the changes Neil Kinnock and his supporters set out to make after Labour's disastrous 1983 election defeat. So Gramsci has been effectively enrolled as a member of the Labour Party and his ideas have been given a new Labourist spin to match". (Milne, 1987, p21).

2 Public expenditure, the welfare state and economic crisis

Much casual discussion about the issue of privatisation assumes that its origin is to be found in political ideology and in the different interests articulated therein. This suits the purposes of those arguing from the left because it allows them to claim that it is doctrinaire thinking that is responsible for the current state of the NHS. Similarly, the right can accept this argument because, for them, the problem with state bodies such as the NHS has been their political refusal to allow market forces to operate.

As a result the debate about privatisation has been left at the level of a conflict between opposing values and philosophies. Consequently, the very real economic problems of the welfare state that underlie the implementation of privatisation are effectively ignored. While accepting that privatisation has a very real ideological and moral character, it is the argument of this chapter that it is first and foremost an economic phenomenon; that in other words privatisation is a response to the difficulties faced by the British economy during the 1980s. The main problem that privatisation has been utilised to deal with is an expanding level of public expenditure in a society with a low rate of industrial growth or with uncertain prospects. Privatisation must therefore be understood as an economic phenomena shaped by ideology rather than an ideological one shaping the economy in its own image.

By accepting this argument it is more easy to understand the processes that affected ancillary workers as they faced up to privatisation. This in turn will help us to realise the inadequacy of a strategy that saw opposition to privatisation as mainly a question of creating alliances and influencing public opinion.

This chapter will begin by examining the debate over public expenditure which has been preoccupying governments and economists for the last decade. It will be established that all schools of thought identify public expenditure growth as a significant problem: the right because it undermines the natural operation of market forces and undermines freedom; the left because it represents a drain on the surplus available to the capitalist class; and the centre because it is inefficient. This will provide a base for situating the development of privatisation within the United Kingdom.

Chapter 3 will go on to look at how these concerns have manifested themselves in government policy. This will include a detailed overview of the privatisation of NHS ancillary services looking especially at what has happened to the position of ancillary staff in the course of this process. The chapter will then conclude with a brief history of the development of unionisation within the NHS and the importance of industrial struggles over pay in bringing a about such a high density of membership. Chapters 1, 2 and 3 will provide the political and economic background for the empirical sections of this study.

The context of the debate about public expenditure

The starting point in the debate over public expenditure is the identification of its tendency towards growth. State expenditure, whether in welfare states or in ostensibly free market economies, has risen considerably since the war. Taking all the OECD countries, government expenditure has risen from 27% of GNP in 1955 to 32.5% in 1969. In the 1970s, just as the world economic recession was developing, the share of GDP that public spending accounted for rose even more rapidly; from 34.4% in 1973 to 40.5% in 1975. By 1981 public expenditure accounted for 45.5% of the Gross Domestic Product of the OECD nations. Britain fully participated in this trend. Public expenditure rose from 32.4% in 1960 to 46.6% in 1975, finally resting at 47.1% in 1981[1].

As was noted above, this growth is not of incidental academic interest, on the contrary, theorists of both the left and the right have seen it as a major cause of economic recession within the world economy. It becomes the real starting point of our investigation. As one commentator puts it:

The argument that the growth of government has contributed to the deterioration of the economy must be of particular concern to those who study or administer the broad set of policies and programmes defined as "welfare" or social policy, for it is that set of policies and programmes which bears special culpability in the new conservative orthodoxy that presumes to explain the secular decline in economic performance. And since virtually every version of that conservative orthodoxy calls for a reduction in the rate of growth, and relative importance, of social policies and programmes, any discussion of the "future of welfare" must examine the proposition that government growth and economic deterioration are causally related.

(Cameron, 1985, p9)

As Cameron goes on to point out, welfare spending bears "special culpability" in producing this deterioration. This in turn has led to the identification by politicians and academics alike of "social spending" as constituting the real content of public spending. This means that whilst much of the debate is addressed as being about public expenditure, what is in fact being discussed is "welfare" expenditure. This is reflected in the fact that many of the analyses of public expenditure have concentrated on the importance of "social spending" to the exclusion of other areas (Gillion and Hemming, 1985; Davies and Piachaud, 1985; Bosanquet, 1986; Klein, 1986.).

This maybe partly due to the fact that many state functions such as the armed forces, the judiciary, the prison service, maintenance of roads etc. are not open to question (although proposals in the 1990s question this. But, it is more likely that it is the result of the immense growth of social spending as both a proportion of total spending, and as an absolute figure. This, in the context of recession, coincides with the widespread belief among many commentators that it is the level of "unproductive" welfare spending which above all else determines the overall economic well-being of an economy. In much of what follows there will be a continual movement between total spending and welfare spending. Welfare spending being the lynch-pin of most analyses of public spending.

Neo-Liberal theories of state expenditure growth

As late as 1976, Rudolf Klein could argue that there were only three models of state expenditure growth[2] and that they only differed from one another in the level of their explanatory focus. Ten years later such a categorisation was flying in the face of reality. By the 1980s writers fell into one of three different "political" camps - either "New Right" (NR), Marxian, or defenders of the social democratic tradition (and this third tradition being very weak)[3].

As it is the NR who have been on the political offensive it is probably best to start with them. To understand their ideas it is first useful to be aware of the fact that they see all economic problems as originating in attempts to interfere with the workings of the market. Their work is as concerned with politics as it is with economics. Bearing this in mind, as good a place as any to start is with Brittan's critique of the work of Downs (1960). Downs' argument was that the level of public expenditure is set by competition between political parties. In his model, each party pursues the policies that it believes will win public support. As spending and taxation are the two principle features of government activity, parties will therefore attempt to turn these activities to their own electoral advantage. This means maximising the visible benefits from expenditure and minimising the visible costs of taxation. For Downs, public expenditure is not as a result of this, too large, but rather it is too small. This flows from his belief that voters are more ignorant about the benefits of public expenditure, than they are about its costs. He concludes from this that the size of government budgets in a democracy can only be less than optimal.

As Klein points out there is little evidence for this argument and little practical logic to it. It treats voters purely as consumers shopping around for the best policies, and thus leaves no room for the role of party ideology. As he argues, the Conservatives do not put a lot of store into trying to win over the votes of Welsh miners (nor does Labourt attempt to attract the votes of property speculators).

Brittan (1975) took up Downs' arguments in his "The Economic Contradictions of Democracy" and reversed them. He concluded that the result of party competition would be to increase the budget above that which was necessary. Implicit in his argument was the belief that there would be a lack of budget constraint among voters caused by their ability to see the benefits of spending but not the costs.

As mentioned earlier this echoes a constant theme of the "New Right", namely that the result of democracy is the "politicisation" of the economy. The argument is most forcefully put by Hayek in his three volume study "Law, Legislation and Liberty" (1973). Here Hayek argues that majority rule "necessarily leads to a gradual transformation of the spontaneous order of a free society into a totalitarian system conducted in the service of some coalition of organised interests" (Hayek, 1973, p2). In this way the spontaneous order of the market is interfered with and public spending increases. Unlike other thinkers who see the increase of state spending as being in the public interest, the "New Right" see in this phenomenon nothing but danger.

The effect of public spending is, according to them, the crowding out of private wealth creation; which then leads to falling output and a rise in unemployment. This in turn encourages expansionary economic policies which start the whole process up again.

In this way the state becomes, or is at least portrayed as, a budget maximising bureaucracy. As Heald (1983) writes "Leviathan, a sea monster, often symbolising evil, has been adopted as the image chosen to convey the dire consequences resulting from an expansion of the fiscal activities of the state" (p270). Following on from this, the analysis of the "New Right" moves to a concern with the system of government. Public Choice theorists such as Brennan and Buchanan (1977) and Niskanen (1971) see the state / bureaucrat as attempting to gain the maximum sized budget. Though they offer different accounts for why this happens (one account sees the process as residing in the state wishing to maximise the excess of revenue over expenditure, whilst the other points to the desires of the state personnel themselves), they all conclude that the process is self-perpetuating. Heald provides a synopsis of this argument as follows:

> Once granted the coercive power to tax, Leviathan will exploit that monopoly power, indulging to the full his natural appetites for expenditure or proclivities for revenue... Once Leviathan has acquired the power of taxation,the citizen (voter/taxpayer) possesses no effective mechanism which can prevent him being exploited by Leviathan. Neither electoral processes in a political democracy characterised by majority rule nor moral constraints deriving from a notion of public duty will constrain Leviathan. The citizens only prospect for limiting such exploitation is at the constitution setting stage when the form and extent of the power to tax is decided and the constitutional constraints on that power are established.
>
> (Heald, 1983, p270-271)

Thus some "New Right" thinkers argue, that not only should there be a strictly balanced budget, but also that there should be the necessity for a two thirds legislative majority for all financial decisions. Hayek even goes so far as to claim that the only hope of resisting the power of Leviathan lies in the creation of 15 year parliaments, limiting the membership of such bodies to those over 45, and denationalising money. "Thus democracy is to be tamed by recourse to a Swiss constitution, the caution of middle age and an immense increase in role for joint stock

23

banks" (Bosanquet, 1983, p17).

Allied to this is another worry that has obsessed the NR; namely the tendency of the modern welfare state to generate expectations among the mass of the population which are then expected to be met. This occurs at the same time as a reluctance on the part of the population to comply with state authority in the form of incomes policies and the like which have been introduced to meet such demands. Consequently, as these demands increase and opposition restricts policy options, the state becomes more and more incapable of meeting them. This results in what has been described as "governmental overload" (Birch, 1984), where the processes of democracy establish demands which ensure dissatisfaction all around.

At a practical level it is very easy to criticise the NR approach. Their Achilles heel is their fundamental starting point; that public expenditure increases of its own accord, propelled either by democratic freeloading, or by bureaucratic pressures emanating from inside the state. Whilst there may be some truth in these positions, at least in terms of small scale analyses of specific budgets, it cannot be an adequate account of the functioning of the state as whole. It is also philosophical speculation of the worst order to assume that public spending is conducted by political parties as a form of mass bribery. If this was true, why not just give the self interested groups the equivalent amount of money, as was done in a much cruder form in the "rotten boroughs" of 19th century England. Another failing of this account is its inability to provide any explanation as to the distribution of state expenditures in terms of specific programmes, or why some (such as provision for the mentally ill), are even funded at all (after all, they have no vote or influence). Even less convincing is the argument of the Leviathan state. The idea that the state's role increases just for the sake of it, is one that removes analysis from the centre of study and replaces it with theology. Nor is this an isolated example; most of the New Right's positions stem from their belief in the inherent "goodness" of the market and the corresponding evil that must come from interfering with it. Thus the analysis lacks any real "macro" understanding of the conditions in which the state operates, and it is on this basis that Hayek can argue for the principle of 15 year parliaments.[4]

The worst fears of the neo-conservatives were realised with the occurrence in the mid-1970s of what Tarschys (1985) has called the "scissors crisis", that is a divergence between government receipts and outlays. It was this change in government fortunes which is charted in the growth of the PSBR of all industrialised nations. Saunders (1985) points out that as late as 1973 there were only six countries among the OECD nations, where total expenditure exceeded revenue. By 1975 there were only four where this was not the case. By 1981 overall deficits existed in all but three countries.

This prompted all sorts of solutions from economists influenced by neo-liberalism. First, in the late 1970s, it was the turn of the monetarists and their identification of the money supply as the root of the economy's problems, but, as inflation came under control (via the effects of the recession rather than through their efforts, see Green, 1987), so their influence waned and expenditure related theories took their place. This was the much vaunted move to 'supply-side economics". Thus calls were made to reduce public expenditure. Among those advocating such a turn was Patrick Minford (1984) who was (and is) in favour of complete privatisation of the economy including the provision of social security. He argued that state expenditure is the most wasteful method by which to achieve "social objectives" because it promotes "inefficiency". Within the sphere of what he describes as "state production", that is the nationalised industries, the tendency to monopolisation ensures that the state has to fund them with more resources than they would require if in private hands. By privatising them, the taxes that pay for their upkeep would disappear and deregulation would lead to a restoration of competition causing the prices of their products to drop. The wholesale de-nationalisation of state monopolies and utilities by successive conservative governments is a testimony to the influence of these ideas.

In terms of the state's provision of "public goods" (the provision of necessary infrastructure etc.) Minford again sees the development of waste. This occurs because the state in providing what are really "private goods" as "public goods" (that is goods only usable by individuals and not the community as a whole) ensures their overproduction. This is because they are provided free of charge and therefore create unnecessary demand. By state provided private goods Minford is referring to the whole gamut of rights to services that exist in the welfare state. In conclusion Minford calculates that this tendency results in between 12.5 and 25 per cent wastage of resources and that public goods should only be provided in cases where the market cannot provide them.

Finally, Minford also points to the way the tax system operates. Here, his assertion is that current taxation policy disproportionately affects two groups of people; the highly paid and the lower paid. This leads to waste because for both there is a disincentive to work harder and earn more. For the rich this manifests itself through a lack of being able to hold on to any additional earnings because of the effects of high rates of taxation. While for the lower paid any extra earned may mean becoming eligible for the higher rates of taxation that middle-income earners pay.

Consequently, the amount of tax revenue that the government could have received is reduced. Minford's solution to the problem is to cut the rate of tax all round and therefore raise the amount of tax revenue.

Minford proposes that privatisation of all but the most essential services is a method, through which the elimination of waste can free resources so that they can "achieve social objectives better" (Minford, 1984, p.xix). In this way the provision of vouchers for education, completely privatised health services (with means tested health insurance complete with no claims bonuses) and the abolition of state pensions would solve the economic impasse faced periodically by the British economy. As he writes in his conclusion his solutions "are essential if the British economy is to regain its dynamism" (Minford, ibid.)

From the vantage point of the 1990s the theoretical vision of ideologues such as Minford can be appreciated. Not only have nationalised assets such as electricity and water been sold off, but so also have low rates of taxation been a mainstay of government policy. Furthermore the introduction of market forces into all aspects of government activity has been notable. The Civil Service has been re-modelled along the lines of semi- autonomous agencies; local government has been encouraged and coerced to put out many of its services to competitive tender and the NHS has seen the introduction of the "internal market" and the separation of tasks between "purchasers" and "providers".

At the same time it needs to be acknowledged that what has been changed has not created "pure" market situations rather, as some commentators have put it, we have seen the emergence of "quasi-markets" (Le Grand, 1990; Bartlett, 1991). These are bounded forms of the market which principally allow competition to allocate resources to competing providers yet still remain in the public sector. In quasi-markets the setting of objectives is separated from the providing of services allowing the state to act as a regulator but not necessarily a provider in an increasingly "mixed economy of welfare". Consequently, ideas such as education vouchers, insurance based healthcare, abolition of state pensions have all remained on the political sidelines while more effective ways of curbing and re-orientating state expenditures have been chosen.

Up to this point we have dealt with theories that are explicitly part of the "New Right". However, there are others who do not share the NR's political or philosophical concerns but whose arguments fall in with their general line of march. In some ways this is a result of the NR's ideological dominance of the area, but in general it is the result of their concern with the tendency towards bureaucratic growth exhibited by the state. The focus of these other approaches is one of identifying the state sector with inefficiency. Unlike the NR they do not blame the excesses of democracy for this state of affairs, rather, they blame the inertia which is built into expenditure plans and the expenditure process (Heclo and Wildavsky, 1981). On top of this is what is termed budgetary incrementalism; the notion that this year's budget is based on last years one. Special attention is given to a narrow range of increase or decrease. As Klein writes: "From the incrementalist perspective, it is the interaction between organisational routine and the inherited pattern of public expenditure that is the key - and the residual problem is to identify the economic, social and political factors which help to influence the gradual modification of the historical legacy" (Klein, 1976, p409).

In concluding this section, what we can say is that the dominant economical perspective (and its many variants) believes that public expenditure is something that must be limited if we are to avoid serious damage to the economy. Within this, the role of welfare spending is of particular concern because of its non- marketed nature and its lack of definable output. Consequently, privatisation and the introduction of competition is an ideological solution to an economic problem rather than purely the expression of an anti-collectivist approach.

Neo-Keynesian views of state expenditure

The period after the Second World War was the era in which Keynesian demand management economics gained the status of orthodoxy in the western world. It was, as a theory, marked out from the theories that preceded it and later succeeded it by its emphasis on the positive role of the state in the economy and its acceptance of the fundamental instability of the market. For Keynes, as for the social democratic tradition that came to utilise his ideas, there was a belief that poverty and unemployment were neither necessary or excusable' in an industrial society, especially one based on democracy. It was therefore the duty of the state to intervene and alleviate these problems. As a result, one of the central features of Keynesian thought was a suspicion concerning the role of markets in the effective allocation of resources - something that had been an article of faith in preceding economic models. The result of this was to use various forms of state intervention to compensate for these deficiencies.

For the Keynesians, state intervention was justified on the grounds that, in a democratic society, the people have the right to expect that certain basic rights will be met; and that the state as their representative will act accordingly. The economic tools used to implement this perspective derive mainly from Keynes' notion of aggregate demand. Here the underlying premise is that the market cannot be relied upon to provide everybody with a job or a satisfactory level of economic growth. This occurs, argues Keynes, because there is a tendency for income not to be translated into spending; rather, increases in income tend instead to result in a growth in savings. This in the context of a growing level of economic productivity will have a long term negative effect on the growth of the economy as firms find they cannot sell their expanded production. Moreover, any drop in income produces an immediate fall in consumption and can turn a minor recession into a major depression.

For Keynes then, the short term effects of a market shake-out, such as a rise in unemployment, will lead to a reduction in spending power and consequently a reduction in the effective demand for other products. This will in turn lead to further layoffs and a further reduction in effective demand. The spiral only ends when a lower level of equilibrium is reached.

In this way, Keynes directly challenged the orthodoxy of free- market economics by claiming that the ethic of abstaining from consumption, far from being a virtue, is in fact a cause of economic problems. Saving is a withdrawal of demand and can only be of any use when it is spent. As one set of commentators write:

> Thus saving is first experienced as a withdrawal of potential demand in the form of money. If producers are conservative and only judge future demand on the basis of present demand then increases in saving will not be interpreted as pent-up demand in the future requiring tooling-up now, but as a loss of markets best met by laying off workers.

(Cole, Cameron and Edwards, 1983, p144)

Consequently, it is necessary for the state to make up for the inadequacies of the market. It must produce effective demand by spending money itself and preventing large amounts of money from being salted away in savings. Cole et al. (1983) argue that at its simplest level this leads to three policy instruments: the government budgetary deficit; the manipulation of the level of interest rates; and the determining of the general exchange rate between domestic and foreign currencies. In order to reduce unemployment the government needs to increase expenditure and decrease income. If there is inflation, then this policy is reversed. The need to control exchange is to ensure that the other two policies can operate effectively.

Under this state of affairs, the economy can be operated in the interests of everyone so long as there is a growth in the level of real National

Income. In order to be able to do this, though, the government needs to be able to increase productivity. This necessitates investment in new machinery on the part of industry. But, unless there are low interest rates it is unlikely this will happen. To solve this, the government intervenes through the policy of its central bank to keep interest rates low. In theory, under a demand managed economy both the interests of industry and of social justice can be met.

All in all, this adds up to the advocacy of increasing the level of public expenditure. And for the 30 years after the Second World War this was indeed the case, as the figures for public expenditure growth cited previously show. Up until the 1970s it was generally believed that economic problems could be overcome by the use of econometrics and that a growth in the level of public expenditure was one way of making this process more efficient.

The situation today is radically different. Keynesianism, as a government policy, has been discredited and the size of the public purse is seen as something to be reduced not expanded. Ironically during the 1980s, the only real advocates of increased public expenditure were those on the socialist left. In the important strategy document "The Alternative Economic Strategy" (AES) published by the Conference of Socialist Economists / Labour Co-ordinating Committee in 1980, it was argued that it was necessary to emphasise the positive case for public expenditure growth, against the common sense arguments of monetarism and not to be frightened of increasing the Public Sector Borrowing Requirement (PSBR). The strategists of the AES aside, it is certainly the case that public expenditure growth is not that popular with policy makers in the parliamentary parties.

The proof of this contention can be judged from the way in which defenders of state interventionism now pose their arguments. Barratt Brown (1984) in describing the Keynesian system claims that its' lack of effectiveness in combating the contemporary problem of stagflation was a direct result of the size of the public sector and the tax drain that this caused. Thus, in a world dominated by multinational companies the expedient device of increasing public spending can no longer succeed; and whilst an expansion of public expenditure was written into the 1987 General Election manifestos of both the Alliance (now Liberal Democrats) and the Labour Party, a concern not to increase tax burdens or to overshoot the growth rate of the economy will probably ensure that neither will enthusiastically endorse expenditure growth[5].

What is interesting about these other views is that whilst they do not share the philosophical presuppositions of the NR, their results are effectively incorporated into the dominant view. This can be seen clearly from the vast (and largely inconclusive) debate in social policy about the extent to which state expenditure acts as a brake on economic growth. The OECD Manpower and Social Affairs Committee's report "Social Expenditure: 1960 - 1990: Problems of Growth and Control" concluded that there was no clear evidence to show that a low share of public spending in GDP is the one and only way to higher growth. Commenting on this report, Klein and Scrivens (1986) point out that there is no need for the welfare state to demand an increasing share of resources. They point to the "fallacy" of the argument that "the Welfare State will collapse if it does not get an ever growing share of an ever-growing GDP" (Klein and Scrivens, 1986, p150). This, they argue, leaves no scope for increasing efficiency and productivity. Similarly, Gillion and Hemming commenting on the same report write: "improving the effectiveness and efficiency of the welfare state is clearly one way of resolving the resource constraint" (Gillion and Hemming, 1986, p167). This statement comes after the expression of concern at the effects of any attempt to use social expenditures as an economic tool to develop the economy. They write:

...across the social programmes generally the magnitude of such positive feed-back effects of increased spending is not likely to equal the first round direct costs. And there are also negative effects on the tax base to be considered arising from higher tax rates, disincentives to work and the emergence of an informal labour market.
(Gillion and Hemming, 1986, p167)

The central problem that affects those concerned with defending the welfare state becomes one of finding ways to reduce expenditure. Consequently, they find their focus drawn to finding ways of providing services in the cheapest manner possible rather than with providing the best possible service. They write approvingly of the "role" of the market in achieving this end. A good example is the work of O'Higgins and Patterson (1984) who point to various methods of reducing growth in the welfare state without having to change it substantially. In terms of specific programmes, Bosanquet (1985) suggests a greater use of informal carers and volunteer staff as well as the recruitment of more skilled employees in the social services to overcome the problems of resource shortage. Judge and Knapp (1985) writing about the relative merits of public and private provision of residential homes for the elderly have this to say:

It is quite possible that in many instances public services could be produced more efficiently if they were contracted out to small private enterprises, but it is equally likely that in other instances this will be impractical. The crucial point, whether or not privatisation is possible or desirable, is that all agencies which assume responsibility for the production of welfare should adopt as far as possible what appear to be the critical efficiency- generating characteristics of small owner-managed enterprises.

(Judge and Knapp, 1985, p149)

While they can all argue against the "rhetorical attacks of those opponents of big government who, armed only with ideological cliches and a few simple bivariate correlations..., attribute the deterioration of the economy to the growth of public spending in general and social spending in particular" (Cameron, 1985, p21), they themselves end up succumbing to its force. A strong indication of this is the embracing by public policy specialists, of the practicalities of implementing market reforms (eg Knapp (1988), Davies (1988), Bartlett (1991)). What seems to have been abandoned above all is the notion of public expenditure growth as a tool of social policy. In concluding this section, what we can clearly point to is a convergence of opinion in non-Marxist economic circles that state expenditure has got to be reduced, and that the introduction of the market is the most effective way of doing so. The NR has made much of the running because, for all their theoretical antedeluvianism, and nostalgia for "laissez faire" social policy, they at least realised that there was a crisis in the economy, one that demanded drastic solutions. The theoretical insolvency of all varieties of Keynesianism is shown by their inability to put forward any convincing solutions to these problems and in their shift in concern towards the supply-side of the question of economic growth.

Marxist theories of state expenditure growth

The concern of this section is to examine how Marxists have viewed the question of public expenditure. Given that this thesis is informed from a Marxist perspective, it will be as concerned with the implications of the theories advanced as with their conclusions. The ideas of different commentators will be placed in their theoretical and political contexts. This differs from the approach adopted in the previous section, in that, there the concern was to see how mainstream thinking had come to see public expenditure as a problem. In this part of the chapter our concern is as much the political consequences of the ideas as they relate to political strategy, as with their implications for public expenditure growth.

Marxist interest in state spending differs from the neo-Liberal and neo-Keynesian approaches described earlier because it is essentially concerned with the replacement of capitalism by socialism. For Marxists, the functions of the state are of concern to the extent to which they help or hinder this process. Viewed in this light, two elements need to be stressed. Firstly, there is the concern to discover what exactly the state spends its revenue on, and why? Secondly, Marxists are interested in finding out what effects public expenditure have on the continuation of capitalist relations of production. The central focus for analysis becomes the existence of the state itself, and not just merely its fiscal and monetary role. Inevitably therefore, Marxist analyses depart somewhat from the methodology adopted by mainstream commentators.

In "The State and Revolution" Lenin was at pains to argue that the reason all states come into existence was because of the irreconcilability of class interests. The state exists, and was created, to ensure the dominance of one class over another. Accordingly, the state's primary function is repressive.

If, however, this was the total extent of the argument there would be little need to study state expenditure itself in any depth; because all it would show us is that state expenditures are all directly related to the use (or potential) use of force. The very existence of institutions such as the welfare state militates against this conclusion. Noting this, Barker (1978) has pointed out that most Marxist discussions of the state have concentrated on this "political" dimension, and have thus tended to ignore other functions. Frankel (1978) goes even further and argues that "Lenin's concept of the state has hung like a piece of stunning stage scenery which obscures the complex machinery backstage. In exposing the repressive apparatus of the state he has bequeathed revolutionaries an insight into the possible reactions of a class under threat, but little understanding of how the bourgeoisie dominate when firmly in the saddle" (Frankel, 1978, p9). The role of public spending and the creation of the welfare state have not, as a result, been dealt with fully, and even when they have been evaluated the analysis has tended towards over-simplification.

From a different standpoint, Mishra (1984) has argued that Marxist theory when forced to come to terms with the existence of the welfare state, first of all did so by addressing itself to a functionalist account of the benefits that accrued to the capitalist mode of production from the existence of state provided welfare. Only more recently has it come to concern itself with the role that the welfare state may play in the destabilisation of the capitalist economy.

Analysis of public expenditure from a Marxist perspective must focus on the dual nature of the welfare state in capitalist societies, as both a stabilising and a destructive institution. As with most most Marxist analysis the two are not only connected but the latter is dependent on the former.

Legitimation, reproduction and stabilisation

As George and Wilding (1976) point out, Marxists from Laski to Miliband have always seen the provision of welfare as a reform offered by a ruling class in order to placate subordinate groups and thus maintain their control over them. The spending of state revenues on welfare is seen as a mechanism for the maintenance of social stability. Public expenditure from this perspective is a necessary cost for capitalism; one which must be taken up to ensure that capitalist social relations are not challenged. Historical evidence relating to the founding of various forms of state welfare is given to support this view. For example: Bismarck's intention in creating the world's first state social insurance system in 19th century Germany was primarily to undercut the support for the then revolutionary Social Democratic Party (SPD). Similarly, Balfour's 1895 comment that 'social legislation is not merely to be distinguished from socialist legislation, but is its most direct opposite and its most effective antidote" is also seen as acknowledgement of the fact. More commented on has been Quinton Hogg's (1947), the later Lord Hailsham's, argument for the establishment of a welfare state in Britain after the Second World War on the grounds that: "if we don't give them social reform, then they"ll give us social revolution" provides evidence of the fact that even in the twentieth century these considerations were voiced.

Discussion of a more precise nature within Marxist theory can be traced back to the intervention of the German Capital Logic school in the 1970s and their subsequent translation and take-up by English speaking writers[6]. Here the concern of Marxists moved from an interest in the legitimating functions of state welfare to the role of the state in providing essential services for capitalism. The focus correspondingly moves to public expenditure as a whole rather than just its social functions.

The Capital Logic school starts it analysis from the belief that Marx's "Capital" is not just a work of political economy, applicable only to the economic level of society, but rather, it is also, an analysis of the structure of class conflict in capitalist society. Because of this, it can be used to understand both the nature of the state and the provision of welfare. Muller and Neususs (1978) argue that because capital can only exist in the form of individual capitals, the state must exist as a separate institution, apart from the competing capitals, in order to reproduce the needs of capital as a whole. It exists to fulfil the needs of capitalism as a system. As they write: "the state is a necessary form alongside and outside bourgeois society", which if it did not intervene would destroy its own basis - the labour power of workers. In this way, it is argued, the functions of the state are concerned with making good the deficiencies of private capital and with organising individual capitals into a viable body. Altvatar (1978) delineates these functions into the following schema:

a) To provide an infrastructure.
b) To establish and guarantee legal relations.
c) To regulate conflict between capital and labour.
d) To safeguard the existence and expansion of total national capital on the world market.

Similarly, O'Connor (1973, p7), whose work we shall return to later, divides state functions into the following three categories:

1) Social investment which "consists of projects and services that increase the productivity of a given amount of labour power and, other factors being equal, increase the rate of profit". This is termed by him as "social constant capital".
2) Social consumption which "consists of projects and services that lower the reproduction costs of labour and, other things being equal, increase the rate of profit." This he terms 'social variable capital"
3)   Social expenses which he argues "consist of projects and services which are required to maintain social harmony". These include welfare expenses.

In their various ways both Altvatar and O'Connor have provided the necessary basis for a more detailed examination of the welfare state from a Marxist perspective (even if they do suffer from an excess of functionalism). Whilst the Capital Logic school have developed their critique theoretically (see Holloway and Picciotto, 1977), others, including O'Connor, have sought to ground their analyses at a more practical level. Ian Gough in his 1977 paper on state expenditure used O'Connor's schema to describe what exactly the state is compelled to do. He too divides state functions into three groups: the first is what he calls military and associated services; these are the armed forces, the police, the judiciary and the servicing of the national debt. These he regards as luxury consumption for the capitalist class.

The second category he terms the social services: these include income maintenance, education, health and welfare and certain aspects of housing. These are all regarded as inputs into the production of labour power. Finally, there are what he terms infrastructural services and economic aid. As he writes: "collected together in this category are those expenditures which either (a) finance state provided means of production or, (b) directly assist private profitability and accumulation. The first group can be further divided into infrastructure expenditures and public corporation investment" (Gough, 1977, p77).

By infrastructure expenditures Gough means: posts, roads, water and sewerage, industrial estates, environmental and pollution control services, urban renewal etc. Public corporations on the other hand produce (or used to) commodities for the market, but, as many of them are what could be termed "basic inputs" for industry, their role again, is to help the private sector. Within this model we can see that the principle role for the welfare state is as an input, via labour power, into capitalist production. These ideas are summed up by Gough in his "The Political Economy of the Welfare State"(1979) where he argues that the welfare state is characterised "as the use of state power to modify the reproduction of labour power and to maintain the non-working population in capitalist societies". Within this role occurs, what we have earlier identified as, the legitimating role of the welfare state. This role is premised on the concept of hegemony; namely that it is easier to maintain the conditions for the continued operation of capitalism through the consent, or at least the grudging acceptance, of the majority of the population, than it is to do so by the straight forward use of force. Thus, the institutions of bourgeois democratic rule are ones that stress equality before the law and representation in decision making. The idea being that the political circumstances under which people live are freely chosen and of their own making.[7]

Part of this process has been the creation of welfare states, or at least the state funded provision of welfare services. As Navarro (1978) reminds us, these are often the result of struggles waged between classes and not just the automatic outworking of an increasingly technocratic capitalism. Thus, to borrow T.H. Marshall's idea, the ideal of "citizenship" is given concrete meaning. Along with the duties and responsibilities of an individual in society goes the right to be looked after by that society. In this way legitimacy is increased. This view has been challenged by the CSE state group (1979) who argued that the state's functions go much further than just legitimising capitalism. They argue, that the state actually creates and reinforces the social relations that are the basis of capitalism. As they write:

Therefore, when we speak of the role of the state in the reproduction of capital, we must remember that we are speaking not simply of performing certain material functions for capitalist industry but of reproducing a certain form of social relations. More simply: what makes the state a capitalist state is not so much what it does as the way in which it does it. For example, any society would have to educate workers for industrial production: what is particular about capitalist education is that it reinforces the atomisation on which class domination is based under capitalism. The state in capitalist society is a class state by virtue of the fact that it deals with people as free and equal individuals, but it groups these individuals in all sorts of ways - as voters in geographical constituencies, as social security claimants, as litigants, as parents, as patients, as taxpayers, etc. However, unlike pre-capitalist class societies, it never deals with people explicitly on the basis of their class position, it never distinguishes between exploiter and exploited.

(CSE state group, 1979, p18)

The work of Claus Offe (1974) also points in this direction, he argues that alongside the "political administrative system" lies the economy and the "normative or legitimation system". This latter system creates a flow of "loyalty" to the political administrative system. This leads to conflicts between commodification and decommodification as the state has to reconcile the conflicting demands of the two systems. As Fitzpatrick points out: "The capitalist state is constantly faced with persistent problems in its three subsystems, with regard to fiscal resources, administrative rationality and mass loyalty" (Fitzpatrick, 1987, p230). This approach allows Offe to concentrate on the particular strategies adopted by the state to overcome its dilemmas, namely; the need for purposive rational activity in the context of its failure to have achievable goals and the ultimate ineffectiveness of decentralised decision making. Offe also points out that further difficulties derive from the need for a loyalty creating "consensus" in areas such as health care which often has to be resolved by "scientizing politics" through the use of experts and the elevation of non political forms of decision making.

In this way the activities of the welfare state are even more fundamental to the well being and stability of capitalism. A fact that increases the importance of political struggle within and over the state.

The welfare state then, as Peter Leonard (1979) has written, is involved in the production of the required quantity and quality of labour power through education, public housing, health, and social services. However in doing so it modifies the structure of capitalist society both economically and politically and it is this tendency to modification that brings us on to the second feature outlined above, namely the possibility of the welfare state destabilising the capitalist economy.

Destabilising and crisis inducing tendencies of welfare states

We have seen that from a mainstream Marxist perspective the functions of a welfare state are ones that interconnect with other parts of the public sector in order to benefit capitalism as a whole. As far as this goes then, the rise in the size and influence of the public purse is seen as unproblematic. For James O'Connor and Ian Gough, the process is not so simple. While it may be the case that overall the welfare state operates to maintain capitalist relations, it can also be the case that the provision of welfare places a considerable burden on the profitability of capitalism. Public expenditure has the consequence of destabilising the system it is attempting to aid.

It is from O'Connor and his seminal "Fiscal Crisis of the State" (1973) that most of the current argument in Marxist circles about the negative effects of welfare spending have their origin. O'Connor's thesis is that while the welfare state exists to assist accumulation and legitimise class rule, the two functions are not necessarily supportive. He contends that the welfare state as a legitimating institution for capitalism plays a major role in slowing down its overall rate of accumulation.

O'Connor argues, in a similar vein to Bacon and Eltis (of whom more later) that there is a "tendency for state expenditures to increase more rapidly than the means of financing them". Hence we get the "fiscal crisis of the state". The reason O'Connor gives for this growth is that the state, in carrying out its accumulation functions is not equally sensitive to all sectors of capital because, among other reasons, the state is not equally dependent on revenues from both sectors; namely the monopoly and the competitive. The state's ability to finance accumulation and legitimation policies depends disproportionately on tax revenue received from both capital and labour in the monopoly sector.

This is because to fulfil the state's basic functions, it must ensure unimpeded accumulation in the key monopoly sector. The relationship between monopoly capital and the state is not, however, asymmetrical. The increasing social character of monopoly production requires a scale of investments that is financially prohibitive, or entails too great a risk for even the large monopoly sector firms to undertake. Only the state has the necessary economic resources and political entitlement to ignore short term profit criteria for such massive investments. The monopoly sector thus actively courts certain forms of state intervention. This is because monopoly accumulation and growth depend upon the continued expansion of state expenditures which are used to socialise investment and consumption. O'Connor concludes, therefore, that not only does the monopoly sector grow by virtue of its ability to shift its costs of production and investment onto the state but, conversely, "the general effect of monopoly sector growth has been the growth of the public sector. In other words the growth of monopoly and state sectors is a single process".

However successful, accumulation in the monopoly sector creates a separate set of contradictions of its own. This is because potential industrial output of the monopolies outpaces the demand for monopoly products. What occurs in these circumstances, then, is the creation of surplus productive capacity, which in turn, introduces systemic tendencies towards stagnation. This brings about the possibility of a realisation crisis, with its attendant promise of disaccumulation, as well as leading to an expansion of the pool of surplus labour. Thus in the absence of significant state activity, stagnation and unemployment become plausible scenarios.

The state cannot afford to let this happen, because, as has been pointed out above, monopoly sector growth is a prime determinant for both social cohesion and legitimacy. Additionally, argues O'Connor, surplus labour power generates political pressure for action by the state and in so doing adds problems of legitimacy to already existing economic problems. O'Connor seeks to argue that state expenditure is forced to rise given its close dependence on the monopoly sector. The work of Griffin et al. (1983) bears this thesis out, at least as far as the U.S. experience is concerned.

So far, what we have been presented with is an analysis that is heavily functionalist in orientation[8] but which doesn't seem to depart much from what previous writers have written. The move that O'Connor makes is to see the tensions that exist between the public and the private sectors of the economy as ones that ultimately lead to crisis. To do this O'Connor utilises an orthodox Marxist account of the way in which capitalism operates. How he does so is explained in an article published in 1981 where he writes:

"Fiscal Crisis" was based on two major theoretical departures from orthodox Marxism's treatment of the state budget. The first was the treatment of certain state expenditures and material activities as social capital, or social investment/social consumption, or social constant capital/social variable capital. This concept of social capital permitted me to study both the quantitative and qualitative meanings of certain kinds of state interventionism. Quantitatively, social capital "ceterus paribus" raises the rate of exploitation, hence the average rates of profit and capital accumulation. Qualitatively, however, social capital "pollutes" capitalist production relationships insofar as transport, education, health services, and so on are organised by the state and hence are not based exclusively on exchange value criteria. In sum, the first theoretical departure was to treat certain state expenditures as social forms of capital advanced, or capital costs, not as revenue drains on surplus value.

The second departure from orthodox Marxism was the treatment of other state expenditures as "social expenses". The concept of social expenses is perfectly consistent with orthodoxy in the sense that both "state revenues" and "social expenses" are deductions from surplus value and thus form a barrier to capital production in that they help solve the problem of capital realisation.
(O'Connor, 1981, p44.)

Thus it is the trade-off between social capital and social expenses that determines the success of state intervention. This is known as the "return flow". If this return flow is not providing an adequate return for whatever reason, then, a fiscal crisis of the state will occur. This simply refers to the ability of capitalism to reproduce itself adequately. On top of this, there is also the the need for capital to be realising a sufficient surplus If this isn't happening then even a positive return flow will cause crisis. O'Connor puts post-war American society in the context of the return flow and its relation with the accumulation of capital in the following passage:

The post World War II solutions to classical overproduction crises (consumer credit, mortgage debt, welfare and the social wage, and other trends and policies designed to underwrite capitalist product competition and the commodification of needs) have stretched U.S. capitalism to the point of capital underproduction. Specifically, thanks to the growth of private consumption and social consumption, from the standpoint of both the size and value content of the consumption basket, there is insufficient production of of inflation free surplus value. And because of the growth of of social expenses, including military and law and order expenditures, there is a larger unproductive drain on the surplus value that is produced. In short, in my view, the general economic crisis must be itself explained partly in terms of the social forces and political struggles leading to the fiscal crisis of the 1960s and 1970s.

(O'Connor, 1981, p49)

To summarise, O'Connor is arguing that both the state's attempts to improve accumulation and its' need to provide legitimacy bring about severe problems for the maintenance of capitalist form of production. O'Connor's method of accounting for these problems is one, which as the final section of the above quotation suggests, is very dependent on subjective factors. By this I mean the role of class conflict. O'Connor has even gone so far as to dub his approach to the economic crisis "workerist" because of the importance it attaches to class struggle. He plays down what he describes as the functional aspects of the crisis. As he writes:

...in my view, the falling rate of profit is not rooted in overproduction of capital (as traditional Marxism maintains) but rather underproduction of capital. The underproduction of capital emerges when the combined demands of both organised and unorganised sectors of the working classes results in a dramatic growth in the "average individual consumption basket" (or the average amount of wage goods workers can acquire with their real wages); an excessive growth of the "value content" of these goods; a concurrent growth in the social consumption costs organised by and through the state; and, finally, when the value content of these social costs rise dramatically. "Underproduction of capital" results when these factors combine during a period when labour power is immobile and inflexible. and when capital has a relative difficulty in mobilising variable capital (or surplus value producing capital).

(O'Connor, 1981, pp41-2.)

This is important to our investigation of the causes and effects of state spending because it seems to suggest that a considerable part of the cause for the economic recession lies with the existence of the organised labour movement. Here the trade unions' ability to extend the legitimating function of the state pushes it to the point where it becomes antagonistic to the existence of capitalism as a whole. Thus we have come full circle; far from the state merely organising the reproduction of labour power, it now acts as a drag to further capital accumulation and is the principle reason for the system's instability. The full extent of this approach can be illustrated by looking at the work of Ian Gough. Here the potential contradictions which are latent in O'Connor's work become more visible as Gough tries to locate his analysis in both a fiscal crisis model and a complementary analysis of the role played by class struggle in determining the recession. This leads him to argue that while at one level there is a fiscal crisis of the state, at another the state is absolved from any guilt. If we deal with the fiscal level first; the welfare state, argues Gough, modifies capitalism by exaggerating the tendency to crisis that is endemic within it. It does so because with the development of the welfare state in Britain there has also been a simultaneous decline in the profitability of British capitalism. Since the 1960s the expansion of state welfare has, in effect, come into contradiction with the process of capital accumulation. This, combined with the existence of a strong trade union movement which has a vested interest in retaining welfare provision and if possible expanding it, has led to both an economic crisis and a concern over the level of public spending:

> Given a low level of productivity growth and the ability of labour to protect real wage levels, it is impossible to increase this growing level of state expenditure in a way that does not worsen inflation or growth or both.
>
> (Gough, 1979, p126)

Even though it is based on a very parochial study of Britain we can see Gough's essential agreement with O'Connor. For him the major source of blame for economic crisis is not the need of the state for more resources, but rather the inability of the state to curb union power. Before we go on to discuss this at a more theoretical level, we first must know how Gough's approach developed because it has some influence on the political dimension of welfare spending.

Gough's arguments were posited in opposition to what has become known as the "Bacon and Eltis thesis". This argument was concerned to identify the drain on industrial investment brought about by state expenditure and was very influential in bringing about the Callaghan government's cuts in public expenditure. It can be argued that Gough in trying to refute the Bacon and Eltis thesis, ends up in a compromised position where his analysis, insofar as it sees state welfare activities as productive, becomes a political weapon to be used against these encroachments[9]. Put simply, the Bacon and Eltis (1976) thesis argued that Britain had a bloated state sector. This was the result of Britain having undergone a process of deindustrialisation since the 1960s which led to a shift from manufacturing industry to the provision of services. The argument is based on the theoretical distinction that they make between the marketed and non-marketed sectors of the economy. The importance of this distinction is that the non-marketed sector is dependent upon the marketed one for revenue. As they write:

> The marketed output of industry and services taken together must
> supply the total private consumption, investment and export needs of
> the whole nation. A difficulty Britain has suffered from since 1961 is
> that the proportion of the nation's labour force that has been
> producing marketed output has fallen year by year, at the same time
> those who have to rely on others to produce marketed output for
> them, civil servants, social workers and most teacher's and medical
> workers, have become increasingly numerous and they have had to
> satisfy their requirements by consuming goods and services that
> diminishing numbers of marketed sector workers are producing.
> (Bacon and Eltis, 1976, pp27-8 quoted in Gough, 1979, p107)

Gough answers this analysis by arguing that in no way does the
unproductive sector incapacitate capitalism's ability to produce surplus
value. This is because taxes, though ultimately paid for out of the surplus
value that capitalism has extracted, do not disappear never to be seen
again, even when the working class consumes them in the form of
welfare. They are not lost because taxes once collected are spent and re-
enter into circulation. Similarly surplus spent on welfare is in fact a
contribution to the reproduction of labour power:

> The value of labour power is thus measured by the private and
> collective consumption of the employed population in capitalist
> economies.
> (Gough, 1979, p117)

As a consequence, argues Gough, the welfare state exists to reproduce
capitalism and not to undermine it. The welfare state's relation to the
current recession then, is not one of cause, but rather one of the
exacerbation of existing problems. However, the conclusion that is
reached from this, is that the state does not bring about dis-accumulation
through expanding its budget. Here Gough seems to depart from
O'Connor.

The question of unproductive labour

At this point in the discussion the question of unproductive labour
becomes important. This is because the extent to which state
expenditures have good or bad effects on the economy as a whole is

dependent on whether or not public workers create value or are a drain on surplus. Gough's argument while capable of dealing with the Bacon and Eltis thesis, means that his work comes into conflict with the Marxian orthodoxy on this question. He does so by challenging the traditional notion of productive labour and its intrinsic connection with the creation of surplus value. The upholders of orthodox Marxism have been universally hostile to his redefinition. They (Wilson (1980), and Harman (1983), among others) argue that Gough's position in relation to state expenditure not only inaccurately reflects Marxist categories but, in fact, flies in the face of them. The hostility between the positions has got to such a point that Elizabeth Wilson has gone so far as to claim that the terms that he has developed to support his view of productive labour (such as "collective consumption", "social wage", "surplus labour" etc.) lead her to believe that analysis has been replaced by metaphor and that his concept of surplus labour is more a journalistic device than an attempt at analysis[10].

To understand the importance of the debate we need to understand the categories developed by Marx. In "Capital", Marx constructed a model of the economy on the foundation that what motivated capitalism as a system was the need to make profit. Profit could only be made by the extraction of surplus value from the direct producer (the worker) and this could only be the result of an employer engaging a worker to produce commodities and then paying him or her less than his or her full worth. However, in order to realise this profit the commodities produced had to be put onto the market and sold. In this way the productivity of labour is determined by its ability to produce surplus value and thus make a profit. It will be obvious from the above that the production of state welfare has very little in common with this process. Unlike commodity production there is no market, accordingly there can be no surplus value, and so ultimately there is no profit to be realised. In classical Marxist terms, state welfare workers are unproductive.

This is why, to keep his argument consistent to his response to Bacon and Eltis, Gough introduces his concept of social labour. This is done to make labour performed in the state sector productive. This can only be done by trying to make it an equivalent concept to Marx's notion of surplus value. Once this is accepted, state workers who participate in activities that lead to the reproduction of capitalist relations of production create surplus labour. By this he means that these workers do not get paid the full value of the work that they do. Because of the equalisation of the rate of exploitation by the labour market, state activity in reproducing the labour force is productive. It is productive in another way as well, for apart from enabling the capitalist mode of production to continue, it simultaneously provides benefits and services to the working class.

It is in this way that Gough can argue that it is not state expenditure that causes the economic recession. However, if this is strictly true, then it remains to be seen how the state can be responsible for the economic crisis. If, as Gough, is arguing state workers are productive then it is impossible that they are draining surplus away from the accumulation process. Also, it would seem to suggest that governments who cut back on public expenditure are acting irrationally. This, I feel, is unjustified. The central problem then, is the question of productive labour and here I am inclined to agree with Wilson when she writes "neither hard work, nor surplus labour, necessarily create surplus value" (op. cit. p83). This is not to impute that unproductive labour is not subject to the same conditions of utilisation as those employed in the productive sector - it is, and as such, responds to its conditions in much the same way; unionisation, strike action, disputes over productivity etc. As Erik Olin Wright (1978) puts it:

both productive and unproductive workers are exploited; both have unpaid labour extorted from them. The only difference is that in the case of productive labour, unpaid labour-time is appropriated as surplus value; whereas in the case of unproductive labour, unpaid labour merely reduces the costs to the capitalist of appropriating part of the surplus-value produced elsewhere. In both cases, the capitalist will try to keep the wage bill as low as possible: in both cases, the capitalist will try to increase productivity by getting workers to work harder; in both cases, workers will be dispossessed of control over their labour process.

(Wright, 1978, pp49-50)

But there is a difference between the two sectors, and it is linked to the question of surplus value. What this means is that in a time of economic recession, the non-productive sector is more likely to be affected than the productive. This occurs in much the same fashion as uncompetitive units of production being forced out of the market in a recession. No-one would argue that these companies were not productive whilst they traded (even if they were doing so at a loss), but given that the surplus that they were making (or not making) was not sufficient to be able to compete with their more efficient rivals then it was inevitable that they would go under.

Similarly, the reproductive functions of the state are productive to the system in the long run, in that they reproduce the labour force. In the short run they cause a drain on usable surplus. This is of little consequence during a period of prosperity, and can actually contribute to the economic stability of the economy by providing markets. But, when the economy is in difficulty, state expenditures create a burden by diverting resources away from immediate use by companies. Here the argument that these monies will re-enter the economy and promote growth is no solace to firms that need the money immediately. As the capital logic school argue, it is the difference between capital in general and the many capitals. In viewing the question in this way we can get away from the necessity to describe state welfare as productive just so as to ensure that it is understood that it performs necessary tasks for capitalism[11]. This position is summed up well by Fine and Harris (1976):

> What we dispute, however, is the notion that this indirect productiveness of state expenditure invalidates the proposition that the state is an unproductive burden for capital. For in Marxist analysis "indirectly productive" and "productive" activities are qualitatively distinct categories. It is therefore not inconsistent for an activity to be both unproductive and indirectly productive.
> (Fine and Harris, 1976, pp98-99.)

What we see now, and to a much greater degree than with O'Connor, is the contradiction between arguing for a fiscal crisis of the state on the one hand and claiming that the recession isn't the public sector's fault on the other. At the best of times, Gough's work shows a vacillation between the two positions, at the worst there is a usage of one in isolation from the other. Thus in a later view (1983) he argues that there is a link between public expenditure and the recession but that it is not so simple or straight-forward as is believed by the NR. He argues that the Keynesian welfare state has generated new contradictions and as a result of these "it is not possible for state expenditure to rise inexorably as a share of GNP without adverse consequences for its domestic capital" (Gough, 1983, p471). State expenditure, he argues, sets two main limits on accumulation. These are similar to those outlined by O'Connor in that extra inflationary pressure in the economy is caused by the states demand for an increased share of resources and, secondly that, it also interferes with the natural operation of the economy and thus impedes the production of surplus value and profit.

Like those of O'Connor these views can only be sustained by the notion that it is not the falling rate of profit that has created the economic crisis but the relative balance between the classes. Thus, in a more elaborated form than O'Connor, Gough can argue that it is not the unproductive nature of state activities that is the principle villain, but rather the intransigence of the working class. It is they who have eroded capitalism's ability to perform well. As he puts it:

> The seeds of the current world crisis germinated precisely in the preceding "long boom" of the post-war years. This both exhausted the post war potential for accumulation and growth within the post-war world and altered the class balance of forces within the advanced countries. Squeezed between these two sets of forces, the rate of profit has declined and with it the motor force for continued growth. The need on the part of capital is to re-establish conditions for profitable accumulation, but the very balance of class forces makes this difficult to achieve unless and until they altered.
> (Gough, 1979, p136)

Criticisms of the "Fiscal Crisis" approach

For Gough, as for O'Connor, it is not the tendency for the rate of profit to fall (TRPF) that dictates the condition of the economy but the class struggle. This position, accordingly, has come under attack from more orthodox Marxists. It has been described by Fine and Harris (1976) as neo-Ricardian in its outlook in that it concentrates almost exclusively on the circulation of capital and not on its' production. In this, they argue, Gough in particular is following the explanation given for the economic recession made by Andrew Glyn and Bob Sutcliffe in their "British Capitalism, Workers and the Profit Squeeze" (1972) and whilst O'Connor is probably not directly influenced, his stated sympathy with the position is enough for the same points to apply equally to him also. Glyn and Sutcliffe argue that the origins of the crisis lie in the simultaneous occurrence in Britain of high wage pressure and an increase in competition within the world economy. Because of this situation, increased wages could not be passed on in the form of price rises and thus they led to a reduction in profits. This view is accordingly popular with O'Connor and Gough because it allows them to argue the case for the primacy of the "Fiscal Crisis" and its attendant emphasis on class struggle. If, however, TRPF has been abandoned for an emphasis on class struggle, it is not just the case of Marxist orthodoxy being offended that is important. Rather, what stems from this decision is the placing of the welfare state in the centre of the stage of economic and political life rather than at its margins. This occurs, because, if economic crises are the result of the competition for resources between capital and labour, then the existence of the social wage (in the form of the welfare state) is a primary area of conflict. Moreover, it therefore becomes essential for capital to reduce its size so as to be able to raise the rate of profit (by indirectly cutting "wages"). If then, we follow through the consequences of O'Connor's and Gough's theoretical decision, we could end up in a position where it is necessary for capital to attempt to destroy (not restructure) the welfare state. Obviously this is not a conclusion that either of the two writers come to, but, it does provide an explanation why there has been so much talk of the "dismantling of the welfare state".

However, to challenge the theoretical starting point of O'Connor and Gough we can cite the response of Harman (1980) who points out that the argument put forward by Glyn and Sutcliffe and also by Rowthorn[12] is both theoretically and factually wrong. The rate of profit did not fall until after the 1970s. On top of this, argues Harman, there does not seem to be any mechanism provided by either Rowthorn or Glyn and Sutcliffe to account for why such an upsurge of wages at the expense of profits should occur, except for the notion that the reserve army of labour had dried up, which was again untrue. In fact the labour market witnessed the entry of large numbers of women and immigrants into the labour force. At a theoretical level the criticism levelled against the neo-Ricardians is that they treat the struggle over the distribution of values between capital and labour as primary. As Callinicos (1982) has pointed out this is very far from Marx's own view:

> The tendency for the rate of profit to fall is bound up with the tendency for the rate of surplus value to rise, hence with a tendency for the rate of labour exploitation to rise. Nothing is more absurd, for this reason, than to explain the fall in the rate of profit by a rise in the rate of wages.
>
> (Marx, 1973, p421n)

Again following Marx, "the rate of accumulation is the independent, not the dependent variable, the rate of wages is the dependent not the independent variable". Callinicos goes on to argue that "the class struggle is not the explanans but the explanandum, it is the phenomenon which itself needs explanation, not the principle in terms of which explanations are made". Thus whilst it is true that exploitation is already class struggle, it is also more than that:

> Marx's theory of crises serves to specify the complex objective conditions not only the relations of exploitation, but the competitive

struggle between capitals - which provide the objective framework within which the struggle between capital and labour unfolds, not to reduce all social relations to mere expressions of this struggle.
(Callinicos, 1982, p158)

Thus it is argued, a properly Marxist account of the genesis of crises must start from the economy and not from class struggle. It cannot be the case that the money spent on the welfare state is the principle reason for the economic crisis. Furthermore, the whole political importance of the welfare state as the pivot of social struggle is thereby reduced. Instead, what is argued is that economic crisis develops out of tendencies that are internal to capitalism itself (such as the TRPF) and that workers struggle and the fiscal burden created by the welfare state merely accentuate these difficulties. For orthodox Marxism then, there can only be political solutions to these economic problems.

However, it is not only on a theoretical and historical level that the fiscal crisis position can be criticised. At a political level the effects of these ideas can be felt too. Firstly, it can lead to the suggestion that all that is necessary for the restoration of profitability in an economy is the shifting of resources from one class to another. In this way, a Marxist justification for a wages freeze can be created. Secondly, and probably more interesting for the purposes of this research, it can lead to arguments about the need for an ideological campaign around issues such as the NHS given the crucial role they play in maintaining the living standards of the working class (and in more general terms the whole population) through the social wage. This does not necessarily mean that being influenced by these ideas leads to the adoption of a position akin to that of the "New Revisionists". But, these ideas can provide a theoretical justification for the importance of such a strategy. This may be especially true if in the light of the current vogue against economism their ideas are interpreted as support for a radical trade off between welfare and wages in a new "social contract". Ironically then, what starts out as an endorsement of working class militancy can in the circumstances of the 1980s, end up as its opposite. Thus, for O'Connor and Gough, the welfare state plays a major part in determining the economic well-being and political struggles of any society that possesses one. The "fiscal crisis" account of the effect of welfare spending on capitalism is one which can only lead to the conclusion that the central struggle is over the provision of the social wage. As we have seen, this may lead to unintended consequences that remove it far from its desire to support working class struggle.

A Marxist account that may be preferable to the ones on offer is one which tries to bring together all the positive aspects of each of them. That is, it sees state welfare as being involved in providing capitalism with an adequate labour force, as creating a certain basis for legitimation and at the same time costing capitalism resources which could otherwise be used for accumulation. In other words, what we are describing is a contradictory structure. Therefore, the precise form taken by this institution will depend on what is the most dominant factor in any period. In a period of stability the reproductive functions will be primary; while, in a crisis it will be its drain on usable surplus that will be paramount. No one single aspect of the welfare state is its entirety[13].

On top of this, we must also be aware that neither the beneficial nor the negative effects of welfare spending entirely account for policy directions. Following Offe all that can be said is that both the positive and negative aspects of welfare spending set up pressures that can be accepted or ignored. Not all advanced capitalist societies have welfare states and not all welfare states are privatising their services.

If we can conclude this Chapter by saying anything, it is that the welfare state does act as a restraint on capital accumulation but not in the way that the neo-Ricardians would have us believe. It is not the central cause of the problems of capitalism but acts as a running sore when the system is not confident of continual prosperity. Thus, we get to a point where Marxist analysis converges with that of the NR. Consequently, it is the case that all major schools of thought see the growth of the welfare state as problematical for capitalism. This leads governments, whatever their hue, to rethink the question of how to provide services to the mass of the population. How it is done does matter given the ideological connotations that policy forms carry with them. The over-riding principle is that it should aim to be done at a smaller cost to the exchequer or reduction to the rate of expenditure increase.

What therefore needs to be emphasized as a result of this, is the economic foundation to to the process of privatisation. As I will go on to show the history of the 1970s is marked by various attempts to curb the rising level of public expenditure. Privatisation is merely one way of achieving this end. The next chapter reviews the development of government concern about the level of public spending and shows how this has generated pressure for privatisation within the NHS.

Notes

1. Figures from "OECD Annual Accounts and Economic Outlook, No 34", quoted in Saunders, (1985, p6).

2. Klein differentiates these three general approaches to the question of expenditure growth as: (a) the societal system approach, (b) the political system approach, and (c) the governmental system approach. These modes of explanation are ordered on the basis of their level of generality. In the first group are those that try to explain trends in public expenditure by changes in the societal system. In the second are those that concentrate on the political system and the role of party competition and ideology. In the third are those that look predominantly at the role of government and in particular at the influence of civil servants.

3. See Heald, (1983, chapter 11), or in terms of the welfare state, Mishra, (1984).

4. A fuller discussion of the inadequacies of the neo-liberal position is contained in Mishra (1984) pages 53-64.

5. An illustration of this is the decision by the Labour Party to divide its 1987 election commitments into two parts; one set comprising of 'priorities' which are carefully costed so as not to place additional strain on the economy and another set which would only be implemented given the availability of resources. This approach has been taken ever since in Labour policy pronouncements.

6. Both Holloway and Picciotto (1977) in their introduction to a collection of essays by German writers, and Jessop (1982) pp90-97 give accounts of this school.

7. This is not to suggest that this was a totally conscious policy on behalf of the capitalist class. But as in most things it was a useful result. For a fuller discussion of the relationship between capitalism and the democratic state see Jessop (1984).

8. And possibly Keynesian in its emphasis on demand management. There are also other problems associated with this approach, namely its distinction between monopoly and competitive sectors. However in terms of the argument that I wish to concentrate on - the need for the state to create the conditions of production and reproduction for capital they are unimportant.

9. Indeed this is the position reached by Freeman and Vandesteeg (1981) where they sum up the political problems of the Marxist attitude to productive labour in the following terms: "The traditional Marxist view cannot really challenge ruling class ideology since it arrives at very similar conclusions as to what is unproductive labour. When the state says that the Health service is unproductive the traditional Marxist theory agrees. We are left with a moral defence but without a critique of bourgeois theory to underpin it" (Freeman and Vandesteeg, 1981, p95).

10. Though to be fair to Gough his position relies heavily on Rowthorn's extension of the concept of non-marketed transfer. This is where private firms (and especially monopolies) extend their operations vertically in the market by taking over companies that provide them with factors of production. The workers in the firms taken over no longer produce for the market but for their owning firm. They accordingly produce no direct profit and accordingly no surplus value.

11. These ideas have been developed from an article by Freeman and Vandesteeg (1981) who point out that Marx has two definitions of productive labour: the first is labour employed by the individual capitalist and the second is labour employed in augmenting of capital as a whole. They argue that the latter definition should be better titled "Marx's description of how the capitalist class defines unproductive labour". This is because it uses the bourgeois notion of profit making as its benchmark. They, like Gough, reformulate productive labour to include state welfare activities but exclude profit making concerns such as private schools on the basis that they merely profit-takers, in that they merely take no role in production and just drain off the surplus produced elsewhere. But if we return to Marx's two definitions we can avoid this conclusion and still see the importance of state welfare in terms of the needs of the economy as a whole. In effect we end up with four categories: 1; (productive labour producing commodities) 2; (unproductive labour involved in the circulation of commodities) 3; (unproductive labour producing services for the working and non-working population) and 4; (unproductive labour producing luxury / non essential items and services that are drains on surplus - private schools, arms production, expensive jewellery etc.) Also see Barker (1978, pp 25-27), and Callinicos (1983a, pp 87-93).

12. Rowthorn writes "...the rate of profit did not fall because the organic composition rose, but because the share of output going to profits fell" (Rowthorn, quoted in Harman, 1980, p47).

13. O'Connor and Gough come closest to this point of view, but their insistence on the fiscal crisis overshadows their insights.

3   Constraining expenditure and the National Health Service

...public expenditure is at the heart of Britains economic difficulties. Higher output can only come from lower taxes, lower interest rates and lower government borrowing.

(1979 Expenditure white paper, HMSO, 1979, Cmnd 7746, p1)

At the centre of all governments' difficulties since the mid-1970s has been the problem of curbing public expenditure growth and (for them) the linked question of inflation. This has affected Labour and Conservative administrations alike. At its most strident it has taken the form of the neo-liberal monetarist economics of the Thatcher governments, but it was also the motive force behind the Healey expenditure cuts of 1976. If we look at the different government's records in turn, what we discover is that while each has tried to deal directly with the problem of state expenditure growth, they have all failed. This is in spite of quite genuine cuts in spending during some periods (the Wilson/Callaghan government of 1974-1979) and in some programmes (housing and education under the two Conservative administrations of 1979 and 1983).

Pliatzky (1982) argues that Edward Heath started the quiet revolution against public spending with his application of the philosophy of the "Selsdon Man" to economic policy. By applying it, the Heath administration of 1970-74 was seen to be attempting to "roll back the frontiers of the public sector and create a social market economy". But with a growth in the unemployment figures and the debacle over both Upper Clyde Shipbuilders and Rolls Royce Aerospace, it was abandoned. Instead, there was a return to long term public expenditure growth as signalled by the November 1971 white paper. So fast was the turn around that Peter Jay was prompted to ask why they had gone to all the fuss of talking about curbing public expenditure in 1970 when by 1972 they were exceeding all of Labour's plans for expansion. Thus public expenditure as a proportion of GDP rose from 36.3% in 1970 to 42.2% in 1974[1].

Why did this happen? Part of the explanation may lie in the fact that the economic problems that faced Britain during this period were not then as serious as those that were to face future governments. But even more important was the fact that the Conservative government was not prepared to break with the post- war consensus that decreed certain macro-economic solutions to the problems of the economy. Thus the "Barber Boom" and increased public spending. Central to all of this, was the need to plan the economy based upon the development of tripartism in which the agreement of the trade unions as well as the employers was essential. This was to be achieved by the carrot and the stick. The carrot of the growth of public services and the stick of the Industrial Relations Act. As Mullard points out: "The growth of expenditure during the period 1970 to 1974 was attributable to the Heath government's acceptance of the post-war settlement. This represented the administration's recognition that they could influence the level of employment and that the rising inflation needed the consent of strategically located groups to control costs" (Mullard, 1985, p192).

In contrast, the Labour government elected in 1974 came to power with the intention of increasing public services and not cutting them back. But by July 1975 a "cuts" package was agreed to, which resulted in expenditure falling below the level that they had inherited in 1974. In 1976 Dennis Healey, the same politician who proclaimed that he was going to squeeze the rich so hard that the pips would be heard to squeak, announced that volume planning was to be abolished and replaced by cash planning as a way of cutting rising expenditure. This was to set the pattern for the following years. By 1979 public expenditure (as a proportion of GDP) had fallen 6.5% below the 1974 level. In terms of specific programmes; housing declined by 34% from 5.08% of GDP in 1974 to 3.31% in 1979, the capital component falling by 59%. The Health budget grew minimally during these years in contrast to the periods preceding and succeeding it. It grew as a proportion of total public expenditure from 11% to 11.84% between the years 1974 and 1979. The Labour goverment was able to hold down the growth of the health service partly through reductions in capital expenditure, which fell from 0.34% of GDP in 1974 to 0.26% in 1979, and partly through the nil growth of current expenditure (a factor that was the result of inflation and the low wages of many health workers). By 1979, all progammes except for Social Security and Health and Personal Social Services had been reduced. Between 1974 and 1979 public expenditure had fallen by 1.05% of GDP.

Why had the Labour government taken this course of action? Again, the answer lies partly in the circumstances in which it found itself. The recession that had begun to develop following the Oil Crisis of 1973 and which was exacerbated by the two Sterling crises of 1975 and 1976 forced the government to go to the IMF. But this in itself does not explain the particular route taken by them. What was of prime significance was that a particular ideological battle had been won, a battle about the nature of public expenditure. This change of view was formally acknowledged in Callaghan's famous speech to the 1976 Labour Party conference. In it he outlined why public expenditure had to be cut;

> We used to think that you could spend your way out of a recession and increase employment by cutting taxes and boosting government spending. I tell you in all candour that this option no longer exists and insofar as it ever did exist it injected a higher dose of inflation and a higher level of unemployment. Unemployment is caused by pricing ourselves out of jobs quite simply and unequivocally. This is an absolute fact of life which no government, left or right, can alter.
> (Labour Party, 1976, p188)

A formative influence on these views was the work of the previously mentioned Bacon and Eltis whose views on the "crowding out" of industrial investment by state expenditures became accepted wisdom in the cabinet[2].

Like the previous Conservative government, central to the Labour administration's concerns was the consent of the trade unions. This they got through the medium of the "social contract". However, unlike the Conservatives, this consent was to be used to drive through cut-backs. Not for Labour the carrot and the stick, but rather the donkey whacking itself. Trade unions had to accept that the era of trade-offs between wage restraint and public expenditure growth had ended. Not only that, they also had to acknowledge the right of the government to reduce spending even if this meant a deterioration in public services. All in all, the government was chasing the notion of a much reduced public sector. In spite of the overall reduction in public expenditure, it was not enough to bring back prosperity to the economy; and as this was the rationale that had led to the strategy being adopted in the first place, it can be safely written that the government had not yet got spending under control.

This brings us quite nicely to the election of the Thatcher government in 1979. Here, the work of analysts such as Stuart Hall (1978) has made popular the notion that Thatcherite Conservatism represented a fundamental break with the past. Not only was it the embodiment of authoritarian and reactionary ideas, but it also regarded the welfare state as an anathema to be destroyed[3]. At the level of popular mythology the government was seen to be determined to do away with such popular institutions as the NHS and make every individual responsible for his or her own welfare.

While there was some truth in this analysis, like all impressionistic accounts it suffered from oversimplification. The conversion of all the leading figures in the cabinet to one or another form of monetarism by the time they were given the opportunity to take office certainly meant that certain economic policies were more likely to be favoured than others. However, much of what they did was an extension of the policies of the previous Labour government. If they broke with the post-war consensus, it was only in the way in which they related to the trade union movement, refusing to let it get involved in the government's day-to-day decision making - a role that the trade union leadership had become used to under Wilson and Heath.

While it is certainly true that the government made no attempt to reflate the economy, at the same time they did not directly challenge many of the established vested interests such as subsidies on trade, transport, agriculture etc. Neither did they attempt (until their third term of office) to alter the funding of the NHS or public sector education[4]. Even more importantly and despite strenuous efforts to the contrary, public spending as a proportion of GDP rose from 39.4% when they assumed office to 43.8% in 1983; an 11% increase in budget. In terms of the health service budget its rate of growth was even faster than that of the rate of growth of GDP; 4.67% in 1979 to 5.32% in 1983; all-in- all totalling a 14% increase in budget and allowing health to grow from 11.8% of total expenditure to 13.2%. Even in terms of the different outlays there was growth. The amount spent on capital projects rose by 0.5% of the GDP (compared with a fall of 0.08% between 1974 and 1979). This meant that 26 hospitals had been completed, and 49 were under construction by 1983. Even the current expenditure budget increased from 4.36% of GDP in 1979 to 4.84% in 1983. O'Higgins and

Patterson (1984) argue that in the period 1978/79 to 1982/83 public expenditure grew in cost terms by more than 6%, all this at a time when economic growth was negligible.

The importance of stating these facts is not to absolve the Conservative government of any complicity in trying to reduce public services[5], but rather to show that the Thatcher administration was not hell bent on an unconstrained ideological crusade as many have made out. Thatcher governments did have a particular ideological slant on the problems confronting the British economy, however, they dealt with them in much the same way as other governments have. What links together the Heath, Wilson / Callaghan, and Thatcher governments is that each of them tried to restore the profitability of British capitalism by increasing productivity at no additional cost to the amount spent on wages. Each in turn failed. As they failed they were forced to make what savings they could in other areas to offset their failure. The Heath government faced with a strong labour movement and a limited crisis fared worst and had to increase public spending. The following Labour government reaped the effects of this failure and imposed substantial expenditure cuts. The Thatcher governments also failed to restore profitability to the economy as a whole (as opposed to the financial sector) or to control the rate of expenditure growth.

Even though the Conservative governments came to office with the idea of reducing expenditure rather than finally resorting to it as happened previously, the pattern remained consistent in terms of how they turned a policy commitment into practice. Within the public services the considerable pressure to reduce expenditure growth and to generally cut back is often implemented in the form of a reduction in manpower and / or wages. The reason why it is labour that is chosen to bear the burden of governmental attempts to curb expenditure lies in the existence of what is known as the Relative Price Effect (RPE). According to Judge (1982), the social services, through the existence of the RPE, accounted for three quarters of the growth of public spending between 1951 and 1983.

What then is the RPE? The RPE is the rate of price changes in the public sector when compared to the private sector. It is based on the assumption that the pay increases of public sector workers cannot be offset by productivity gains. Thus within the NHS, a pay rise for nurses cannot be offset by increasing the ratio of patients to nurses unless it is agreed to reduce the quality of service. The whole theory of the RPE stems from the work of Baumol (1967) who argued the familiar position that the economy is made up of two parts; a progressive sector and a non-progressive sector. In the progressive sector productivity increases offset rises in wages while in the non-progressive sector, due to service delivery's labour intensive nature, this is not the case. As there is a tendency for wages to rise in tandem in both sectors the rate of increase in the non- progressive sector will therefore tend to be higher.

Gough (1979) extends this analysis by arguing that because of the critical role played by labour costs, the RPE only applies to state provided services and not to transfer payments from the state to beneficiaries. He also claims that because of the problem of measuring productivity within the social services, independent of the numbers employed; "an alien capitalist logic" is inscribed on "a sector of the economy which is shielded from the operation of the law of value, or market pressures" (Gough, 1979, p85). The consequence of this, he argues, is to assume that productivity is directly related to the total output divided by the numbers employed.

This immediately means that the question of curbing welfare expenditure growth is one of reducing the workforce and their total wages. It was probably this fact that lay behind the decision of the DHSS to "cap" the manpower levels of the NHS in 1984. This was well understood by commentators examing trends at the time. The analysis of O'Higgins and Patterson (1984) made in the early eighties expected even more pressure to be placed on the workers in the welfare services. They wrote:

> When the results are examined across all the scenarios then, it is clear on our fairly conventional assumptions about expenditure pressures and changes at the detailed level, public spending is going to rise in real terms over the next decade. The magnitude of the rise ranges between 6 and 9% in 1988/89 and 11 and 19% by 1993/94. From a starting point of 41% in 1988/89, the scenarios show the programme expenditure/GDP ratio between 38% and 41.5% by 1988/89 and 35% and 42% by 1993/4. The central prospects for public expenditure are therefore for slow growth, accompanied by a decline in the share of GDP for which it counts.
>
> This suggests that it is unlikely that the government's stated target of zero real growth in public expenditure during its current term of office can be met on current policies.
>
> (O'Higgins and Patterson, 1984, p31)

Built into this hopeful analysis of the development of state spending (the authors were of the mind that a public expenditure crisis could be averted given a reasonable rate of growth) there was the assumption that public sector wages would increase more slowly than those in the private sector. However, even O'Higgins and Patterson have to admit that this is not an entirely plausible argument even if it had been true of the years previous to their comments.

They calculated that if public sector wages rose at the same rate as those in the private sector (2.5% per annum in real terms) then real public spending would rise by about 3.5% faster by 1993/94. In the long term this would, they argued, result in a roughly similar programme expenditure/GDP ratio (37.5 to 36.3% in 1993/94), but what it meant in the short term (i.e. the mid to late 1980s) was that given a government committed to keeping expenditure as low as possible it was more feasible to slow down the rate of increase of wages rather than to cut budgets in any wholesale way.

In this light, even the nominal figure of a one percent efficiency saving every year in terms of the cost of inputs every year would result in large savings.

..whilst real public expenditure increases by more than 5 and 10% over the five and ten year periods respectively on the conventional assumptions, the addition of the efficiency gain assumption reduces the growth to 2% and less than 4% over the comparable period....This efficiency gain assumption therefore has twice as great an impact on the results as the change in the wage comparability assumption (i.e. keeping public and private sector wages equal). As argued earlier, if there are no efficiency gains in public services then we do face difficulties in financing public services which provide good standards of service to consumers, and good levels of pay to producers.
(op.cit. p34).

If we ignore the contention that rises in productivity will result in a raising of pay, what we are presented with is the fact that that NHS staff were about to (and did) encounter a period of acute financial pressure which of necessity resulted in job losses and increased workloads. However, not all sections of the workforce faced this pressure equally. The NHS management structures ensured that those working in an ancillary capacity fared worst.

The NHS and the squeeze on expenditure

If we accept that state expenditures on social services in the UK increased during the 1970s and 1980s, where does this leave our analysis of the NHS? As I have tried to point out above the very pressure of economic difficulty forces governments into trying to limit expenditure growth by whatever means possible, and this in general means limiting the expenditure on staff costs. The privatisation or contracting out of ancillary services in the NHS came to have an importance out of all proportion with its savings. Before we go on to look at privatisation in more detail, it is, perhaps, first useful to look at how the government's concern with curbing expenditure growth affected the Health Service up until the mid 1980s. Gough (1979) suggests that the government has dealt with its problems in the following ways:

> We have noted, then, four ways amongst others in which the state, acting in the long term interests of capital, may seek to restructure the welfare state at a time of economic crisis like the present: by adapting policies to secure more efficient reproduction of the labour force, by shifting emphasis to the social control of destabilising groups in society, by raising productivity within the social services and possibly by reprivatising parts of the welfare state.
>
> (Gough, 1979, p141)

Whilst the first two objectives outlined above are not directly relevant to the NHS (though the concern in cutting the length of stay in hospitals etc. certainly fulfills the first objective), the second two have very direct relevance. In terms of raising productivity, several policies have been implemented during the past few years. Firstly, under the Health Service Act of 1980, health authorities were now legally required to keep within their cash limits. Secondly "efficiency savings" were introduced by central government as a means to restrain expenditure. Authorities were expected to find 0.5% of growth money from within existing budgets. To ensure that this occurred the same amount was deducted from their budget allocations. Since 1984 health authorities' efficiency savings have been euphemistically known as "cost improvement programmes". Thirdly, reductions in the numbers employed in the NHS were requested in September 1983, and though not repeated they set boundaries for the setting of budgets. Fourthly, in the changes in NHS spending that were introduced after the 1983 General Election, the RAWP policy of equalisation of resources by differential "growth" was transformed into a policy of equalisation on the basis of differential "cuts".

Finally, the underfunding of pay rises to doctors and nurses in the NHS by the government meant that authorities had to find the finances to pay for them out of other budgets, thus playing off against each other, patient and employee.

The introduction of moves to restructure the delivery of health care reflected the New Right's critique of the NHS as being bureaucratic, inefficient, lacking clear objectives or the knowledge of how to attain them. The 1982 reorganisation of the health service which had the effect of making the District Health authorities the main operational tier of the service was a reflection of this process, as was the introduction of "performance indicators" as points of reference in the assessment of service activity. The Griffiths Report of 1983 was a further step in this direction. Its recommendation for the introduction of general managers, on short term contracts at all levels of the NHS, but especially at unit level, was intended to facilitate rapid change within cash-limited budgets. Ironically, it was this budget consciousness among NHS managers that led to the NHS crises of the late 1980s where the need to keep within budget led to the closing of facilities and to an ensuing public outcry. It also led to the "NHS review" and the acceptance of competition between hospitals as the best way to allocate resources.

In terms of Gough's final category, that of privatisation, there was also considerable movement during the 1980s. The most important (at least for this study) was the privatisation of ancillary services, however, a number of other changes also occurred. One was the steady erosion of the notion of free provision of services at the time of use. According to Mohan (1986) prescription charges had risen by over 1000%, and the price of NHS lenses by 300% by 1985. The general free supply of NHS glasses was ended, with glasses only being paid for to those who passed a means test.

Moves were also made to make the private sector stronger (by relaxing constraints on it) and to link up the NHS with the independent sector. The Health Services Board which was set up by Labour in 1976 to supervise private hospital developments was abolished and consultant's contracts were relaxed permitting them to undertake more private practice without it affecting their state salary. The effect of this was to allow whole-time consultants an increase in the amount of private work they could do.

The linkage between the private and state medical services that the government wanted to encourage is illustrated by a 1981 circular that notified health authorities that they should "take account of the current and planned facilities available in the independent sector" when they planned their own provision. Moreover, the previously existing restriction on the contracting out of patient care to profit-making hospitals was also removed.

The privatisation of NHS ancillary services

As has been written above, of all the initiatives in the NHS taken by the first and second Conservative governments the implementation of privatisation was the most significant as well as the most contentious. It has been seen as the culmination and embodiment of the political changes that swept the country. However, it is also seen as essentially political in character. It is the purpose of this section to look beyond this view and reiterate the economic foundation to privatisation. In so doing, I shall be emphasising the material effects that privatisation has had on ancillary workers, effects which provide them with reasons to be opposed to it.

As Laurance (1986) points out it is not just the fact that private firms were doing government work that is central to the importance of privatisation; domestic services in the Ministry of Defence had been successfully privatised at an earlier date with little concern voiced. Rather, the question that is raised is the fundamental one of the form in which health care is provided, and who is to be ultimately responsible for its provision - the individual or the state. As he puts it: "The country does not give a fig for the state of the country's army barracks, but it cares very deeply about the state of its hospitals" (New Society, 18th July 1986).

Because privatisation is an issue that embodies in a symbolic form all of the piece-meal changes that have occurred to both the NHS and the welfare state since the election of the Conservatives in 1979, what we are presented with is the dominance of the ideological form over its content. One commentator sums this up when he writes:

"Privatisation" is a word invented by politicians and disseminated by political journalists. It is designed not to clarify analysis but as a symbol intended by advocates and opponents of the processes it describes to dramatise a conflict and mobilise support for their own side. Thus it is a word which should be heavily escorted by inverted commas as a reminder that its meaning is at best uncertain and often tendentious.

(Donnison, 1984, p45.)

However, to understand its operation in the NHS we must go further than the rhetoric. We must clarify what is specifically meant by privatisation. The best definition of the term is given by Heald (1983) who points out that there are 4 different components that together can be described as making up the concept "privatisation"; these comprise "charges", "contracting out", "denationalisation and loadshedding", and "liberalisation". Though diffuse in terms of function, what all share with each other is a "strengthening of the market at the expense of the state" (Heald, 1983, p298.). It is in this way that such an "umbrella term" covering many different policies can be regarded as a strategy. A strategy that operates through its component parts in order to restructure the balance of the economy (see Yarrow (1986) for an overview of its significance for the economy in general).

At one level the driving force behind these strategies is ideological, is the need to "liberate enterprise and enthusiasm" (Posner, 1982, p32.) by reducing the role of the state and increasing consumer choice. In this it owes a great theoretical debt to Hayek and to Friedman. But sooner or later the ideological proponents of privatisation do admit to the financial choices that provoke such strategies. In terms of the second and third categories of Heald's model, Peacock (1984) writes:

> The choice between using directly employed resources and resources supplied by private contractors has always existed in the UK, but it is only recently that pressure has been put on central and local government departments, notably through the cash limits system of expenditure control, to adjust the balance towards outside contracting, as a means of reducing costs whilst maintaining the standard of service.
>
> (Peacock, 1984, p4.)

He goes on to explain this away by claiming that since then, at least at the level of government policy, there has been a shift away from talk of savings to the taxpayer (read in government, as until 1987 the promised lower rates of taxation, that were supposed to result from the introduction of the market never materialised, except for those on high incomes) and a move to the importance of competition as a principle. This in many senses is not the argument that it first appears, rather than a principle triumphing over financial concerns, what has occurred is the same objective being achieved by different means. The privatisation of concerns such as British Telecom, or the profitable parts of BL etc. did not in any way increase competitiveness, they merely transferred ownership and raised additional revenues for the treasury. In this way, all the different forms of privatisation are linked together by common concern with the financial crisis. This is as true of the NHS as it is of cuts in the housing budgets. To quote William Laing (1982):

Health authorities have, since the inception of the service, been free to contract out their services more or less as they please. This discretion applies equally to general or "hotel" services, such as cleaning, portering, laundry, catering, and so on, and to patient services such as pathology, diagnostic tests or even operations. But contracting out has remained a relatively rare exception to the in-house rule.

What makes it a live issue now is the conjunction of two phenomena: a Conservative Government strongly committed to privatisation, together with a funding crisis in which cash- limited authorities are being forced for the first time to look critically at how they spend the bulk of their money, not just at the margins.
(Laing, 1982, p25)

He concludes that "the primary advantage from using private contractors should be cash savings". For the DHSS the fact that the amount spent on cleaning hospitals ranged from £200 per 100 square metres to a figure of £3000 was reason enough to entertain the idea. Similarly the cost of cleaning 100 articles ranged from £5.90 pence to £17.60 pence. Another factor influencing government thinking is that of being able to shed responsibility for staff by no longer having to directly employ them. According to the Sunday Times (20th January 1985) the Government aimed to save £100 million from privatising cleaning, also it has been estimated that sick pay and holiday pay accounted for 14% of the NHS wage bill, pensions another 21%. As Coyle points out:

The Government opened the way for contractors not to provide these benefits and therefore the possibility of significantly reducing the £1 billion a year that it costs to provide cleaning, laundry, and catering services.
(Coyle, 1985, p15)

Privatisation then, had its roots in the attempts to curb state spending. The fact that it became the favoured strategy for dealing with this problem is as much a reflection on the bankruptcy of technocratic socialism as it is of the ascendancy of the New Right. Underlying all the rhetoric was the need to save money, but to do it in such a way as to minimise protest. The reason, then, why ancillary services became the

64

main victim maybe because, to adapt an argument of Le Grand's, they neither employed the most vocal sections of society nor did the middle classes directly rely upon them (Le Grand, 1984). This situation can best be seen in relation to another sector affected by government restraint; higher education grants for students. Here proposals during the mid 1980s to change the method of funding students met massive resistance and were quickly dropped. This was mainly the result of the intensity of middle class opposition. Ancillary services did not get such a reprieve. The DHSS circular of 8th September 1983 put it in its proper context. In it Health Authorities were asked:

> To test the cost effectiveness of their domestic, catering, and laundering services by putting them out to tender (including in-house tenders) where these tenders show that savings can be made, a contract should be let.
>
> (DHSS circular 1983:18)

The circular also stated that authorities needed to demonstrate that these services were provided as efficiently and economically as possible. Thus as Paul (1984) points out, the private sector was being offered a potential 3 billion pound market, that is almost one-fifth of the total Health service budget. However this windfall for the private sector would be costly, the whole purpose for the government, after all, was to save money, this could only be found out of the profit margins of the contractors.

There is evidence that the market understood this too. Leading city stockbrokers Laing and Cruikshank concluded in a report on contracted services, that for practical and political reasons, only a limited amount of this potential market was ever likely to be realised.Among problems they envisaged was the opposition of trade unionists and health service administrators who for differing reasons sought to limit the growth of privatisation. Trade unionists in the NHS realised that profits could only be made out of them if they were made to work more productively - this increased efficiency could only come out of their pay and conditions of employment. Whitfield writes:

> The only way contractors can win public sector work is by undercutting wages and benefits and demanding much higher levels of productivity. Employing fewer workers and making them work harder for longer hours reduces costs.
>
> (Whitfield, 1983, p56)

The administrators on the other hand resented the interference of government and private contractors in the running of their institutions and were consequently unsympathetic to privatisation.

The material effects of privatisation on NHS ancillary workers

As noted earlier, the main effect of competitive tendering, whether or not the private sector was been successful, was to put pressure on workers in those areas put out to tender. As the Laing and Cruikshank report makes clear:

> There is the function of the competitive tender itself. This initially encourages the direct labour to pay more regard to its own costs and the quality of its service in attempting to retain business. In Birmingham, for example, the direct labour municipal cleaners retained their position in open tender, having agreed a package with the council which included a 30 per cent reduction in staff and longer working hours.
>
> (Contract Services, Jan, 1984, p39.)

That ancillary workers would be disproportionately affected by this move is indicated by the fact that approximately 85% of the total costs of any cleaning budget are those of labour. As an article in the first edition of "Contract Services" a magazine produced for those hoping to enter the field of privatised services pointed out, the only way in which profits could be made was from the effective deployment of labour, and this in turn was linked to the demand for greater productivity:

> The results of our studies strongly indicate that productivity is a vital factor to be scrutinised by those people who are presently engaged in compiling specifications.
>
> (Contract Services, Jan, 1984, p34.)

This was as true for in-house contracts as it was for privately let contracts. Although an in-house tender competing against a private tender would not have to make a profit, it needed to cut its costs to roughly the same level in order to win the contract. One good example is what happened in one of the health authorities studied. The hospital cleaning services were put out to tender in November 1983 and the original budgets for cleaning two hospitals were £292,774 and £157,728 respectively. The DHA tendered to reduce costs in both hospitals to

£225,084 and £95,422. This resulted in staffing hours at the first hospital dropping from 2,018 to 1,559 and at the second from 871 to 626. Thus even with an in-house tender being successful privatisation has its effects, a total of £4,490 alone being allocated for redundancy payments, each year for 3 years, at just these two hospitals.

This is important to note given that at the time of the study the competitive tendering process was running heavily in favour of in-house bids. According to Laurence (1986) up to the end of March 1986, just under 150 contracts had been awarded to the private sector as against 520 awarded in-house. However, this was a temporary outcome, resulting from lack of competition among contractors, allowing "a handful of companies [to] pick and choose the most profitable plums from among dozens of contracts put out by often reluctant health authorities". He concluded "a buyer's market has become a seller's market" (New Society, 18th July 1986).

The resumption of the advance of the private sector was inevitable given that savings on private contacts were higher than those let in-house. Consequently, when the deadline glut was over and the market settled down, the private firms started to seriously compete again and thereby forced the in-house tenders down also.

It is illuminating to look at the conditions the private firms offered. In the mid-1980's employees of the big three companies operating in the field :- Crothalls, Exclusive, and HHS were all paid Whitley Council rates. However, this situation was a voluntary one reflecting a desire among the major contractors to shake off their "cowboy" image. An indication of its frailty was provided by the government when they abolished in 1983 the "Fair Wages Resolution" of 1946 which protected the low paid. In October 1984, Kenneth Clarke then Minister for Health, followed this up by writing to all health authorities telling them that they should not specify the terms and conditions of service which private contractors should provide for staff working on NHS contracts. As he wrote:

> Attempts to set wage rates and conditions are likely to be against the interests of the Health Authority and its patients because the effect will probably be to restrict competition for contracts and add to any contractors costs.

What is clear from this reply is that the Whitley guidelines constituted a level of wages higher than the government wanted companies to pay, but which in the past they were legally bound to. This in combination with the abolition of most of the existing wages councils put pressure on companies to find other ways to cut wages. The most obvious way was through the erosion of conditions of service. Ascher (1988) points to two ways in which the tendering process has had this effect. The first was the alteration or outright abolition of bonus payments. She estimated that such bonus payments made up between 10 and 25 per cent of a hospital cleaner's basic salary. She writes:

> Before the introduction of competitive tendering and contracting out, authorities were reluctant to attempt adjustments to these bonus schemes; now such adjustments are taken for granted in an attempt to develop a competitive in- house bid. The impact of revised work schedules and bonus schemes upon employees is straightforward: less pay for the same work or more work for the same pay.
> (Ascher, 1988, p109)

The second way in which conditions of service changed was by a "reorientation" of the hours worked by individual employees. Again she writes:

> On average, more than two-thirds of a contracting company's employeees are part-timers and this, combined with skilful scheduling of full and part-time workers' hours, has allowed contractors to make dramatic savings over what might be considered "normal" labour costs.
> (Ascher, 1988, p109)

These tendencies were clearly demonstrated in the health authorities under study. In one not only were the hours worked by domestics reduced, but their entitlement to holiday and sickness benefits had also been considerably altered. Under NHS employment ancillary workers were allowed 20 days of annual leave in their first year rising to 25 days after 10 years service. The contracting company's conditions of employment give workers 15 days after one year and 20 days after 10 years (that the annual leave entitlement does not increase at all after the second year suggests that the company puts little store in trying to keep its staff, or even in regarding them as permanent). Similarly the company have cut the number of Bank Holidays workers can take by 1 day (from 10 to 9). Sickness benefits too, have roughly fallen by a third with payments only extending to 4 months instead of the 6 months offered to NHS employees. An ill worker will get nothing from Exclusive after 8 months, where previously they would have been covered for a whole year, (6 months full pay, 6 months half pay). Whilst the pension scheme offered by the company pays slighty more than its NHS equivalent, it is not inflation proof.

Because during the 1980s reducing NHS ancillary services represented the easiest way to make savings on current expenditure, domestic workers working in the NHS were under tremendous pressure both to work harder and to receive less.

Trade unions, the NHS, and privatisation

Having now outlined the nature of the process of privatisation, it is time to put it in the context of NHS trade unionism. This is important because the material effects of privatisation are only one side of an adequate examination of the situation of NHS ancillary workers, the other side; their organisational response is just as important. Along with the well documented expansion of public expenditure in the post-war period there has also occurred an equally large increase in public sector employment. Not only have the numbers of these employees become greater but also so has their likelihood of being members of an appropriate trade union. As Bain and Price (1980) have pointed out, this has been a constant feature of trade unionism in Britain. As long ago as 1948 the density of public sector unionism was 70.7% as against 37.3% elsewhere. In other words it has remained roughly double the level of unionisation in the private sector, with rates in 1978 being at 81.5% as opposed to 43%.

The expansion of the public sector has not automatically ensured the maintenance of this density. In fact, the areas of most growth have been the traditionally non-unionised areas such as clerical work and other jobs with a high female involvement. What has occurred is a change in the nature of public sector trade unionism, away from the staff association approach and towards a sectional trade unionist stance. Thus since the late 1960's civil servants, teachers, local government officers, and hospital staff have all taken industrial action. In part this new direction on the part of public sector trade unionism is a direct outcome of the new importance attached to the amounts of money spent on paying for these workers. It is no accident that major planks of at least two recent government economic strategies have been concerned with the curtailment of public sector wage increases. The largest increases in the membership of unions such as NUPE, NALGO, NUT etc. have not only come in a period of the greatest growth of public sector employment, but also at a moment of the most intensive industrial conflict.

The NHS has experienced both of these processes, not only coming to employ in excess of a million people, but also having by the late 1970s a trade union density of over 80%. But whilst the NHS has always been a large financial commitment employing large numbers of people, again its density of unionisation was by no means automatic. This density has risen from only 32.2% in 1966 to 73.4% in 1979. This process has been aided by the industrial relations practices of the NHS (the existence of a centralised collective bargaining system operating through binding national agreements etc. such as the Whitley councils), however, the main impetus has come from the desire of health workers to catch up, or maintain themselves, in wage terms with those in the private sector. Thus by the 1970s the downward drift of health service pay that occurred during the 1960s had been reversed by a combination of favourable incomes policy and industrial action. The new found public sector militancy that had contributed to the ending of the Labour government's incomes policy, did not disappear with the election of the Conservatives in 1970. They too brought in (in 1972) an incomes policy, but one which did not give health workers any dispensations and which led to a lowering of their standard of living. The pay of an NHS female ancillary worker fell from 89% of women's average earnings in 1972 to 85% in 1973, this was after increasing from 87% in 1971 (see table 1). For female nurses and midwives their pay fell as a proportion of average earnings from 113% to 105% and then to 98% between 1972 and 1974, for male nurses and midwives the respective figures were 78%, 71%, and 61% (source: new earnings survey, 1985). This pattern was repeated throughout the seventies with health workers increasingly having to take industrial action to keep up the value of their wages, and government incomes policies constantly bringing them down.

To compare trends over the last ten years....The most striking point is a marked cyclical pattern with periods of three to four years of slippage in the pay league reversed by sharp increases. The pattern is certainly consistent with the contention that health workers lose out in periods of strong incomes policy; the erosion of pay coincides with the incomes policies of of the Heath (1972-74) and Callaghan (1976-79) Governments; the catching-up with industrial unrest culminating in outside reviews - Halsbury for nurses and professions supplementary to medicine in 1974, Clegg for ancillary staff, ambulancemen, nurses and professions supplementary to medicine in 1978-79.

(Public Money, December 1983, p62.)

This analysis goes on to argue that "increased militancy may, then, have paid off in securing periodic catching-up settlements, but it has not led

TABLE 1: NHS PAY AND AVERAGE EARNINGS

	71	72	73	74	75	76	77	78	79	80	81	82
MEN												
nurses & midwives	79	78	71	61	na	92	89	80	81	91	91	85
ancillary	78	76	70	78	83	80	78	76	71	79	71	67
WOMEN												
nurses & midwives	113	113	105	98	122	117	113	103	105	111	109	106
ancillary	87	89	85	101	103	97	94	92	86	92	83	83

Source: Public Money, December 1983

TABLE 2: MAJOR STOPPAGES 1971-81

YEAR	GROUP	AREAS	WORKERS	DAYS LOST
1972	Ancillaries	various	94000	94000
1973	Ancillaries	all areas	55000	285000
1973	Ambulancemen	Goole/Bradford	400	5600
1974	Ambulancemen	Glasgow	1000	5000
1974	Prof. & Tech.	Various	1170	136000
1976	Ambulancemen	South East	265	5500
1979	Ambulancemen	Various	6300	34000
1979	Ancillaries	All Areas	n/a	n/a
1980	Prof. & Tech.	Various	10000	2500
1980	Ancillaries	Newport	325	5100
1981	Ancillaries	Manchester	500	5500
1981	Ambulancemen	Various	1300	25000

Source: D.E. Gazette

to a permanent rise in relative pay"(ibid). What this points to then is that the growth of trade unionism in the NHS seems to be closely related to industrial action or, at least, to the contemplation of it (as tables 1 and 2 show when viewed together). As Heald has pointed out in reference to all workers in the public sector: "What is indisputable is that the feeling of being unfairly treated has stimulated unionization as a defensive response and weakened earlier inhibitions against taking industrial action" (Heald, 1983, p211). This has become even more pronounced as expenditure has become a major worry to governments as demonstrated by the imposition of cash limits by all governments since the mid-seventies. Cash limits have as their direct aim the trading off of wage increases for the continued provision of service. An example of this is the way one health authority publically claimed that, as a result of impending pay claims they were going to have to reduce overall spending on services. Heald puts this in the context of recent economic policy:

... the relationship between cash limits and collective bargaining was fundamentally altered by the collapse of the Labour Government's 5% pay policy in the winter of 1978/79. Originally, cash limits had been set by following through the implications of an economy-wide pay norm. Later, the assumptions built into them became the implicit public sector pay policy. For example the Conservative Government used 6% for 1981/82, 4% for 1982/83 and 3.5% for 1983/84 whilst rejecting the idea of a return to an incomes policy. Settlements above these figures would now result in offsetting reductions in volume spending, unless the cash limits were relaxed. The contrast with 1974/75, when volume spending could be maintained irrespective of current settlements, is complete.

(Heald, 1983, p226)

However not all working in the NHS are at the same level or have the same interests. There is a world of difference between the consultant member of the Royal College of Surgeons, and the hospital domestic in NUPE. Thus of the 41 organisations recognised by the Whitley Council for negotiating purposes, 33 were single occupation professional associations. Given that it is these professional associations who held the majority of Whitley council seats (15 to the 14 held by the TUC affiliated trade unions) it is their interests that tended to predominate over those of the others on the council. What is important for the purposes of this study, then, is to separate off ancillary workers from other groups in the NHS. As can be seen in Table 3 it has been the ancillary worker members of NUPE (and other manual unions) who have provided the

TABLE 3: STOPPAGES AT WORK IN THE NHS 1966-1982

YEAR	STOPPAGES	STAFF INVOLVED	DAYS LOST
1966	2	500	500
1961	1	78	200
1968	1	80	80
1969	8	2500	7000
1970	5	1300	6700
1971	6	2900	4700
1972	4	97000	98000
1973	18	59000	298000
1974	18	4070	23000
1975	19	6000	20000
1976	15	4440	15000
1977	21	2970	8200
1978	37	5400	23000
1979	30	635800	1418000
1980	38	6200	179000
1981	35	22900	89000
1982	N/A	180000	781000

Source: Public Money December 1983

backbone of the union's industrial action, without receiving many of the benefits. They have been the ones who have taken the majority of the action in the pay disputes and it is they who faced the brunt of privatisation.

How then did the unions respond or intend to respond to the effects of privatisation? Here the point to be conscious of is the very process that built the union; namely industrial action against government incomes policies (stated or implicit). The 1982 pay campaign though well supported by public opinion got manual workers in the NHS nowhere financially. The form in which the campaign was organised, selective action, limited strikes, and regional days of action involving other unions, was one which squandered the militancy that had been built up and which left those taking part out of pocket and demoralised. When the dispute was finally given up by the TUC leadership at the end of the year, a widespread feeling of hopelessness and apathy prevailed. Neale (1983) himself a participant in this strike, gives the following account of tactics in the strike:

> The one day strike was a success. The union leaders found participation all over the country far more solid than they had expected. On the other hand, the one day strike did nothing to move the government. So the TUC had to find else to do. In the jargon, they had to "step up the action". They decided on more strikes and a campaign to reduce the NHS to accident and emergency cover.

> They called two one day strikes: the first on a friday and the next on the following tuesday. This was a masterstroke. It was more militant than a one day strike. It was twice as much striking. It had exactly the same effect on the government as a one day strike. (two times nothing equals nothing.) It lost the members twice as much money. (two times ten quid is twenty quid.) The TUC was able to step up the action without achieving any thing other than exhausting the troops.
> (Neale, 1983, p92)

Resistance to privatisation, "the cuts", and hospital closures has consequently lacked the dynamism that marked the seventies. This can be attributed to this defeat in 1982. It has meant that the methods of resistance that were adopted, and the ideas used to account for these methods, are marked out differently than they would have been if there had been a victory. This is not to suggest that in the past unions such as NUPE had been officially committed to industrial action as an automatic course of action. Indeed the opposite has been true, with the majority of

NHS militancy in the seventies being of an un-official nature. What may be true is that if that high level of industrial militancy was still a feature of NHS industrial relations, then it would have been more likely that resolutions, such as that at the 1983 NUPE conference calling for coordinated national industrial action against privatisation would be realised, and not just existed at the level of rhetoric.

To conclude, privatisation has had a tremendous effect on the lives and working conditions of NHS ancillary workers during the 1980s. In these circumstances there was a pressure for this group of workers to resist the new conditions being forced upon them, but, given that this pressure followed a period of defeat and demoralisation among trade unionists in the health service, the effects were not uniform and stable. Different groups took different forms of action with differing motivations. However what we can say is that it is these elements that form the "material" basis for any discussion of the ideological struggle that is waged around the issue of privatisation in the NHS.

Notes

1. For an indepth presentation and breakdown of public expenditure trends in the 1970s and early 1980s see Mullard (1985).

2. A Cabinet Working Paper of July 1976 states the following: ".. industrial recovery will be accompanied by the industrial sector seeking funds which will lead to the public sector pre-empting resources or even worse bring a spiral of interest rates which would chasten that recovery" (quoted in Mullard, 1985, p222).

3. This viewpoint is one which is best summed up in terms of the 'crisis of the welfare state'. Its' elements are delineated by Mishra (1984, pxiii). It is the subject of Golding and Middleton's "Images of Welfare" (1983) and is challenged effectively by Taylor-Gooby (1985, 1985a), Therborn (1985) and Mishra (1986).

4. As early as 1982 O'Higgins wrote: "the most radical feature of the recent public expenditure plans, as expressed in the 1982 white paper is the switch to cash instead of volumne planning, rather than any drastic reshaping of the welfare state. In fact... the public spending picture once unravelled shows an almost total failure to convert rhetoric to reality" (O'Higgins, 1982, p154).

5. After all, what is being discussed is the amount spent on these services not on their effectiveness. As Walker writes: "...the public sector may consume increased resources simply to maintain an existing level of services, and at the same time lose ground in relation to the private sector" (Walker, 1982, p5). On top of this is what Gough (among others) describes as the restructuring of the welfare state. This is the process whereby state welfare is adapted to serve the new needs of the capitalist class. According to Gough (1979) this means the switch from the direct state provision of services to public subsidisation and purchase of privately produced ones. Whilst as Taylor-Gooby (1985) has pointed out, this process is extremely uneven, It has resulted in the large scale of council housing (with half a million council houses out of seven and a half million being sold off at up to 40% discount). As well as this, there is now the attempt to put more emphasis on informal care within the community as a way of cutting costs. All in all, There is a complex debate on how far the policies of the present government have affected the provision of service. For an insight into the debate see Illife (1983, 1983a), Robinson (1986) Papadakis and Taylor-Gooby (1988).

4   Ideology and the privatisation of NHS ancillary services: The view from the rank-and-file

This chapter is concerned with describing the opinions towards privatisation held by two interviewed groups of NHS ancillaries in two localities: Health Authority A and Health Authority B. Individuals in both of these two groups were affected by the competitive tendering process and took industrial action in response to it. Both groups also failed to halt the implementation of privatisation. In the course of being involved in action against privatisation all of those interviewed developed some views towards the issue, and towards the government's commitment to it[1]

As outlined earlier, NHS ancillary workers were confronted with a clear opposition between the values of the welfare state and those of the "free market". Unsuprisingly their views fall down very clearly on the side of the welfare state and collective provision. Of course, this might reflect no more than their own awareness of where their own self-interests lay. But what is of more importance is the way that, in the course of utilising these arguments to promote their cause, their own self-interest in winning what is in all other senses an industrial dispute took second place to the question of the "fight to save the NHS". In so doing their ability to succeed in restoring their jobs and conditions was undermined. This connects with arguments raised in chapter one outlined earlier; namely that the input that the strikers received from their trade unions (NUPE, GMBATU) concentrated overwhelmingly on this "ideological" dimension to their situation (pictures of dirty toilets etc.) at the expense of their industrial dispute.

While much was made of the dangers to the public from privatisation little publicity was been made about the erosion of jobs and conditions that privatisation entailed. This is not to say that there was no acknowledgement of these issues by the unions, there was, but it is certainly the case that the emphasis was on privatisation as an attack on the Health Service rather than upon its effects on union members. Consequently, it not suprising to find that the focus the union adopted was one of looking to the general public as a whole for passive support rather than to other unionised sectors of the economy for industrial solidarity. While bearing all this in mind, it is also true to say that there were factors other than the unions' position on privatisation pushing the striking ancillaries to adopt the positions that they did. Among these was the experience of working in a hospital with its attendant caring environment and the quasi-professionalism of many sectors of the workforce.

Rank-and-file attitudes

In presenting the ideas used by NHS ancillary workers to describe their attitudes towards privatisation, the first thing that must be acknowledged is that much of what follows is a synthetic construction on my part. In other words the logic and coherence (or otherwise) of the ideological positions that are articulated is rarely apparent to the person being interviewed. It is the role of the researcher to put diverse ideas together and demonstrate their connection or lack of fit. Whilst this does make interpretation of the evidence of interviews more difficult than would otherwise be the case, it does provide the basis for asserting the contradictory and partial nature of respondents' ideas. For without the lack of definition, the blurring of concepts and the interconnectedness of all their experiences, the ideological contradictions held would become very much more apparent and would necessitate resolution on the part of those holding them.

Domestics in the NHS work in a sector which has one of the worst records of pay and conditions of work. It is a predominantly female occupation (of the 700 000 people working in cleaning jobs in 1985 - 75% were women) and the hours worked are overwhelmingly part-time. Women tend to take these jobs because of the flexibility of the hours that can be worked (i.e. outside normal working hours) and because of the lack of alternative work. Beardwell et al. (1981) in the course of a Low

Pay Unit survey of cleaners in the civil service found that the vast majority of cleaners were between the ages of 35 and 59, married with family commitments, and had previously worked in unskilled employment.

The implementation of privatisation in the guise of competitive tendering represented a further deterioration in ancillary worker's pay and conditions from an already poor starting point. At Hospital A in Health Authority A and at Hospital B in London the effect of privatisation led groups of predominantly female ancillary workers to take various forms of industrial action. All of those interviewed saw the new conditions under which they were expected to work as the main reason for their action. The G&M steward at Hospital B pointed out her hours of service had gone down to four hours a week so that now it would take the whole of a three week rota in order to get her previous pay for a week. As she said:

> It's always been known that hospital workers are very low paid and you either go in liking that sort of work - which we did, or you didn't do it. We didn't get an awful amount of money, in fact we came out very very tired after a days work. But they surely didn't expect us to half kill ourselves for a matter of £20 a week. I mean, really some of us would be coming out with £17 a week ... there's a majority of widows, one-parent families and people with husbands who are out of work or want someone in that hospital for something to live on. Nobody, I defy anybody to live on £20 a week. That is all they were prepared to offer for which they said was casual labour.
>
> (G&M Steward, Hospital B)

Thus in a situation of a 51% reduction in hours and a 46% reduction in costs as at Hospital B, ancillary workers were forced into taking strike action. Again as another G&M member pointed out:

> We didn't want to come out on strike, we would rather have carried on working, but there's no way you could go on working on that wage, you've got to have money to live on, and where there's no money you've got to do something.
>
> (G&M member, Hospital B)

This then can be seen as the bottom line in tracing out the purely economic consciousness of the ancillary worker. It is a response to what are essentially economic pressures. In both Hospital B and Health Authority A it brought about strike action, though of radically different durations. As if to back this argument up, the structure and activities of the workers' trade unions reflected the pace and circumstances of their work. In both Health Authority A and Hospital B the threat of either national strikes or privatisation prompted or pushed some individuals into taking union posts and led to the organisation of meetings, strike activity or pickets where previously there had been little interest. Thus in Hospital B the strike by the ancillary workers against their new condition of employment revitalised, the union leading to a change in the branch officials with the chair - a non-domestic - resigning.

The concerns that operate at this level are ones that are familiar to industrial relations bargaining in every sector of the economy, in that they relate to a desire to maximise the effect of the action against the employer. Following on from this, once the unions had managed to get all their members involved in activity, the main concern was to get support from other unions within the NHS as well as those in the wider labour movement. Here their success was varied, but showed essentially the same pattern. In Health Authority A during both the 1982 Pay strikes and the strike at Hospital A the strikers received support from many different unions and organisations but very little from people in the health service. In the strike over privatisation in 1983 the situation was so divided that ancillary workers at other hospitals in the district only provided the most token of industrial support. As for other workers in the hospitals; the nurses, the clerical staff, the technicians etc. the main response was one of hostility (with the nurses being especially notable in their invocation of ethical arguments against striking). As the NUPE branch secretary in Health Authority A put it, they were willing to go on a march but not to picket. This pattern was repeated at the Hospital B with more support coming from outside groups such as striking miners, Labour parties etc. than from other hospital workers. Even supportive action from other ancillary workers in the NHS was disappointing. There was little response even when other groups of workers started to undergo the processes of competitive tendering. This is not to say that there weren't attempts to coordinate such actions as the attempts by Hospital B strikers to influence their trade union conferences illustrate. But what action did occur was sporadic and in response to local conditions.

In just describing the conditions of trade union activity the emergence of factors which cut across the operation of normal trade unionism and which derive from the institutional nature of the NHS can be seen. This difference is not only represented by the nature of the job - that is working in a hospital - but exists also in the very concept of privatisation; the introduction of private firms into a non-profitmaking public service. That this is important can be seen in the response of one

81

of the Hospital B strikers to the conditions which she found when she moved from another NHS hospital to work at Hospital B, which at that time had already subcontracted its cleaning to an outside company (Crothalls) though at NHS rates:

> When I started here after working in an NHS hospital, I couldn't believe what they were like to work for. They couldn't give a damn, you had to lie to say you had cleaned things properly, a terrible way of going on; whereas if you worked for the NHS theres no need to lie, you've always got everything.
> (NUPE member, Hospital B)

Even in circumstances where it was admitted that it made little practical difference who their formal employers were (and even in Health Authority A the management of the domestics was by a private contractor) they still concluded that "obviously we would like to have been in the NHS" and that private contractors should have been prevented from getting established in the first place. It is factors such as these that move the terms of the ideological debate further away from a purely industrial basis and onto a more political one; one where the ethical acceptability of private involvement in the NHS is raised. It is clear that the issue of privatisation brings into play all of the differing ideas about state provided welfare. The discussion of the workers attitudes and opinions becomes more complicated and confused from this point on.

Part of this confusion can be said to derive from the fact that competitive tendering and the privatisation which normally accompanies it has a drastic effect on the style of work undertaken by the ancillary worker. When asked what they thought of private contractors, it was mentioned by nearly everyone interviewed that what mattered under the new conditions was economic efficiency; that domestic duties were undertaken in terms of the letter of the contract rather than in response to the needs of both cleanliness and the patients. As one Hospital A worker put it "The human element is missing, they're just talking about dirt but its not just that, its people". Thus while it was widely believed that the new allocation of hours made it impossible for the hospital to be adequately cleaned, it was this changed rationale that had the most impact. Again quoting a Hospital B striker:

> We did extras, a lot of extras - that wasn't our duty, we liked the job.... and where we could we ran around for the patients, like getting them soap and buying their papers, but you'd no longer

have time with those sort of hours. Well, its all what working in hospitals is all about; cleaning work is all about helping one another, even if it means staying on to do your own bit of work, because you've gone off the ward to perhaps find a patient a phone. But you won't get that sort of thing now.

(NUPE member, Hospital B)

Part of resentment to this intensification of work is its reduction to what they see as the status of casual work. As a G & M member at Hospital B was at pains to point out, they were "trained, experienced workers".

I defy any housewife to go into a hospital if she thinks its like housework, it isn't; its vastly different than housework, you've got to know what you're doing. Patient care comes into it, patients looked forward to seeing you come in. But he said all that had to stop - the hours he gave us were just for cleaning and not for talking to patients, handing them a glass of water if they wanted it. All that had to go by the board, and to us that was criminal.

(G&M member, Hospital B)

And again:

I worked in a surgical ward for well over 12 years and I knew exactly what I had to do, we had operations every day, and I knew exactly where to go - where it was morning operations when they were to have their tea and what they started off with. And afternoons whether they were to have their tea in the mornings, all that, I knew exactly what I had to do for the operations, you had to know your diabetics, you had to know whether they had sugar, they weren't allowed biscuits, they weren't allowed all these different foods and you just had to know what to give them.

The sisters and the nurses could leave the domestics who worked on the ward absolutely alone because they knew what they were doing, they knew that if a person was going for an operation they wasn't to eat. And after the operation how long they had to go without food and drink. The sisters knew it would be done properly.

(G&M member, Hospital B)

Here the connection between taking action over conditions and pay, the reduction in status and the nature of the NHS as an institution comes together. When the strikers at Hospital B discussed the people who replaced them, not only were they disparaged as "scabs" but they are also seen as people who weren't interested in providing the service the hospital and the patients deserve. A G&M member back from visiting a Welsh hospital where she had been trying to publicise and gain support for the strike at Hospital B spoke of how her "heart ached" to see the cleanliness of the hospital in contrast to the situation she saw existing at Hospital B. Thus contempt for taking peoples' livelihoods away is translated into a sentiment of moral outrage against those putting financial interests above those of the community. In this way the element of the NHS representing the whole community is brought in on the side of the strikers and indeed of any one taking action inside of the NHS against what are euphemistically known as "the cuts" (privatisation comes into this category because of its purpose to save money at the expense of workers).

However, this is not just another level to the motivation of the strikers, it is in reality a different form of strategy. One that exists in a state of tension with the other motivations. This is not to suggest that it is a fundamental contradiction. It can quite easily co-exist with all the other elements because, at least initially, it works in their interests. It allows them to extend their base of support to the whole "community", to present their concerns as public concerns and similarly to argue that the industrial action that they are taking is for the benefit of the whole community. This can be seen in the response to the question "why are you taking this action?" This was the answer of the NUPE shop steward at Hospital B:

> The simple fact is that we care so much about the service we provide that we are actually putting our livlihoods and our time to fight for that service and the overall service in that hospital is not our responsibility. It is the health authorities responsibility and so therefore does the health Authority really care what happens to the patients at Hospital B when they agreed to such a ridiculously low tender put in by the company. Are they responsible people? We're the responsible people, we're the responsible ones, we realise that the service couldn't be provided for the patients at Hospital B. There was no alternative but to take strike action thats why we spent 15 months on the picket line - because we care for hospitals and people.
> (NUPE steward, Hospital B)

As mentioned above, the move to defending their actions in terms of the interests of the community-at-large was not one that was devoid of consequences. It started to affect the activities taken, because once articulated as a principle, the notion of the community-at-large's interest will come to interfere with the specific interests \ objectives of groups taking industrial action. This is a problem that spreads across the whole of the public sector but is probably most acute in the NHS because of the type of service provided. The main problem with this approach is in its "limiting" of the forms of activity that can be "legitimately" taken by the strikers.

As stated before, the main aim of any group of workers in dispute is to put sufficient pressure on their employers so that they are forced to concede whatever is the cause of the dispute - traditionally this is done by disrupting the operation of the institution. However in the NHS if this was done successfully it would, of necessity, mean stopping the operation of routine medical and health care tasks. In the case of Hospital B the strikers first objective would be to close the wards, stop all admissions, move all patients to other hospitals, and stop all out patient services. In other words close the hospital down completely. Whatever the industrial sense this makes, in practice this is impossible. The problem with this strategy is that whilst it certainly meets its objective of making it impossible for the hospital administrators to run their hospitals - this is as far as it affects them. The main impact is made not on the management but on the patients, and the patients represent the whole community given that the NHS exists to provide health care to the whole community. Herein lies the strikers' dilemma.

The consequence of this situation is the unstated limiting of actions by workers in the hope of maintaining (or achieving) the support of the community. This usually ensures that the hospital in which they work functions more or less normally. The explicit reason given for this policy is that those working in essential services "could not take action without jeopardising peoples' lives." The alternatives open to strikers in this sector are thus limited by their own concern not to act in a callous way. Attempts to find out what effect this limitation had on individuals were made by asking them about the limits to their action. A good example of the way that strikers deliberately underplayed their hand is provided by the NUPE branch secretary from Health Authority A, who in recounting the period of the 1982 NHS pay dispute said the following:

> We made it a rule that no ambulance, whether it was an emergency ambulance or an outpatients ambulance was to be stopped, we woudn't stop any ambulance whatsoever. Although one or two that came from London, they did offer not to go

through, and we said no you go through - I wouldn't stop an ambulance because I always look at it, it could be my son.
(NUPE steward, Hospital A)

Similarly, and in direct contradiction to the NUPE steward's claim that they were not concerned with these issues because they were employed by private contractors, is what a G&M member said about the Hospital B strikers' attitudes to effective industrial action:

You can't very well in a hospital - we could have. We were thinking of the patients, we could have stopped a hell of a lot when we first came out - the water board came up and they said how many different unions were in the water board and how every one was for us, and that they would cut the water off completely. Do that and we could have had this strike over in days, but then we said no, and they said what about emergency - just enough - and we said no, we didn't have none of that, we wouldn't accept any of that.
(G&M member, Hospital B)

In what was seen as an attempt by Hospital B management to undermine and demoralise the strikers, an incident occurred where a number of obviously ill and elderly patients were dropped at the picket line with the strikers being told to make a decision about what to do with them. To quote the response of one of the Hospital B strikers "we were all flabbergasted" - decision making of this sort is obviously an area which brings the narrower sectional interests of trade unionists into conflict with the interests of the community (and indeed with themselves as part of that wider community.) As the same Hospital B G&M member concluded:

We done it on ourselves really, we did, we could have ended this a long time ago if we had been hard enough to do it, but we've not.
(G&M member, Hospital B)

To this description of what can be regarded as the industrial and trade union influences on this group of workers must be added the more overtly political dimension of the issue of privatisation. It is this interaction between the occupational and political influences that forms the matrix of this group's ideology or "common sense". As indicated earlier the question of privatisation was linked in most individuals' minds to the perceived erosion (and / or dismantlement) of the NHS as a public health system. A typical comment about what they saw as the effect of privatisation was the following:

> We was the envy of the world, our equipment is second to none, but I think its just going to be drained down and down, and the queues are getting longer. I don't know where the savings are going from these contracts, we've not getting up the queue any higher, I don't know where all the savings are going when all you've got is dirty hospitals... the patients have just got to accept that the hospitals are just not so clean. We did have the best health service in the world, didn't we?
> (NUPE member, Hospital B)

From a male NUPE steward in Health Authority A :

> They want to move to the American style health service... open the market for the cowboys, come in, clean up, disappear.
> (NUPE steward, Hospital A)

In responses to the question asking for the reasons that explained privatisation, there was a strong belief that the processes that led to privatisation were linked to a general political strategy that went beyond health care:

> Maggie Thatcher wants everything denationalised and that includes hospitals, so really she's selling off something that belongs to the public. Everybody is entitled to a clean hospital but the way she's working it its like a two tier system, that's what she wants. This is good enough for the working class; contractors anything - that'd do for them! and the good work is for the private patients, thats no lie, its true, but what the contractors are going to pay these cleaners they're only going to get rubbish in, because only people who do rubbish work will accept that type of thing.
> (NUPE member, Hospital A)

Unsuprisingly, the nature of health provision and the form in which it is conceived, become central to the attitudes and opinions of this group and in turn provides the basis for a moral understanding of the world:

> The NHS will disappear, it's going to be like it used to be - when you want treatment you're going to have to pay for it and that will

be that. If you don't belong to a private health insurance scheme or something, you're going to have be like America - you either pay on the nail - that's what it was like before the war and I think you're going to find people are going to die through not getting any treatment. It's (the NHS) the finest thing that happened to this country, you take before, I can remember my mum and dad doing without when we were kids: did you take one of their doctors or did the rest of you eat, you had a choice and I think thats going to come back.

(NUPE Branch Secretary, Health Authority A)

Two issues become crucial here in producing this defence of the existing make-up of the NHS, they are:
1) the role of profitmaking;
2) the perceived differential class interests in different forms of health care.

On the first issue there were very strong opinions about the "wrongness" of making profits out of the NHS and of the effects of private medicine on the NHS.

No-one should be able to make money out of the NHS like the contractors are making money, it wasn't dreamed up for that type of thing, it was to help the poor people not the rich getting richer - that's wrong.

Of course you're making someone rich. I'd never thought about it like that but being out here has brought it to your mind, we've found out that Tory M.P.'s - Michael Forsyth he's a Tory M.P. - gets thousands of pounds, he's a majority shareholder for Crothalls [a contracting firm]; and Crothalls puts thousands of pounds into Tory party funds every year for their election thing. I mean you don't know all that when you're working for them, you don't know that someone's got their fingers in from the Tory party owning it. Whereas if you're working for the NHS you know its yours and it's going back into the state - state owned its yours.

(NUPE member, Hospital B)

The reasons why the question of profit making is so important is the role it is deemed to play, not only in terms of their jobs, but also what it means in terms of the kind of health provision that is available. Reference is constantly made about the kinds of illnesses that profit making medicine is deemed to be interested in:

> And lets face it, these private health schemes, they don't want the very ill, the terminally ill, they only want the cream, they don't do hip replacements and the poor won't be able to go private - look at Maggie Thatcher; when she had her eyes done the instruments had to come from the NHS.
>
> (NUPE member, Hospital B)

The issue of profit making seems to them to be all about relegating the health of the working class - their health - to a second class status by making it no longer universal and free. Obviously this involves the invocation of principles of an abstract nature, such as collective responsibility for health, the unquestioning meeting of needs etc. But in the main, at least for this group, there are more practical motivations for these attitudes, and interestingly, ones that come from their status as patients.

> Since this privatisations been out, the doctors and all that don't seem to have time for you now because they're only interested in the private people who are prepared to pay. Where before you could go to a doctor, whether you was national health or what and he'd sit and listen to you. It has got a choice now of going private or private patients. He'll do that rather than national health because he's getting more money.
>
> (G&M Member, Hospital B)

That there is an antagonism between the NHS and private medicine is accepted by all. That the purpose of the NHS is to look after their health, and that of private medicine to look after that of the rich is also accepted. It was regarded as quite wrong that there should be any private usage of the NHS whether it was of equipment or of resources such as blood:

> Private medicine should be kept out of the NHS - those that can afford Swiss clinics let them go to Swiss clinics. But, national health is the nation's health, for the majority of people, the masses, not the plutocrats who can afford to drive in the Rolls Royces to have his ingrowing toenails done, let him go private if he wants that sort of care, away. No way should they use beds like that. No! Private medicine has it's place, but not within the NHS. We should be totally devoid of it, because we're actually

89

subsidising it, you and I are subsidising private medicine because, they're using your facilities, your beds, and all they're paying for is the actual surgeons time. It's as simple as that.
(NUPE steward, Hospital A)

If they're private, then they should pay for the blood, people give their blood for nothing, the blood donors and then you're getting people going around making dough on someones blood which they give for nothing. Really, if you delved into it, you'd scream."
(NUPE member, Hospital B)

In making this radical separation between private and public medicine, attempts are made not only to force an absolute division but in some cases to denigrate the quality of private medicine and to generally attempt to promote the NHS by undermining some of the common justifications for the existence and need for a private sector in the NHS:

They reckon that if you're having private health you're taking the work load off the NHS.
[Another voice] That's rubbish because they've got beds in the NHS.
[Original voice] Yeah, and what the doctors doing is making the list longer by going seeing to a private patient, isn't he? Every time he takes on a private patient, the NHS patient he's got to wait another whatever how long and then he might get another, get another private one come along. I mean you'd be seen in a couple of days in a NHS hospital.
(conversation between NUPE steward and NUPE member at Hospital B)

The attitude being alluded to then is that there is near total opposition to private medicine but only insofar as it occurs in the NHS. This distinction is quite important because in many ways what it represents is not a total rejection of the market in health provision, but a limiting of these non-market values to a collectivised health service that serves the interests of the working class / poor. Thus, there is an implicit acceptance of the private sector but it is an acceptance which says it must be totally separate. Further evidence for this view can be gleaned from responses to the question about what they felt about private health insurance. A typical reply was one from the NUPE branch secretary in Health Authority A , "Private Medicine? On yeah if anyone wants it, it's up to them, fair enough if you've got the money" or that from a G&M

member at Hospital B:

> Yes if they've got the money they're entitled to do what they like with their money as long as its kept out of the NHS. Build another hospital, another clinic if they've got that much money. Doctors charge enough for these private patients to go see them, leave our national health alone.
>
> (G&M member, Hospital B)

As if to illustrate the limited nature of the non-market ideas that form some of the basis for the opinions of this group; when asked how they would like to see the NHS improved, only those with the most trade union experience such as the trade union officers gave much scope to the possibilities of workers control or indeed of socialism. The overwhelming viewpoint was that what was needed was a massive injection of money and the removal of governmental interference in the running of hospitals.

In other words what was being sought was a return to the previous status quo in which the NHS existed, and in which the values of equality and free care for all were supposed to exist.

> I think the national health should be free and that's all you should need. I think the whole country should be national health, but the only thing is the waiting list - that's the reason people pay, they can get it done quicker. This isn't what was meant by the health service... I'd like to see it expanding, not deteriorating like it is at the moment, bigger hospitals,better hospitals, more wards that's the type of thing that you need. You want more hospitals not less. You've got a bigger population so it stands to reason that you need more and the better the health service was the longer people were living.
>
> (NUPE steward, health Authority A)

This is not to suggest that everything should be left as it was. It was also generally acknowledged that. "it isn't run as efficient as it could be" and that this must entail cuts of one sort or another. However, it was felt that the fault lay in the misuse of facilities and the growth of administration.

> Nye Bevan, he intended a health service where you'd be healthy from cradle to grave, it's not worked like that mainly through the amount of immigrants that have come in. He did intend Britain

to be healthy and it would pay for itself. He didn't forsee immigrants and disease, I just don't know where the money goes.
(NUPE member, Hospital B)

Half thats wrong with the health service at the moment is that theres too much administration talking about growth and development - the only thing that's developed in [Health Authority A] anyway, is the administration. I think you've got more administration than all the others lumped together. I really do, if you go up there and see how many offices and how many buildings are taken over by office workers and honestly half the time you go in there and all they seem to be doing is a lot of paper work and at the end of the day, its all in the bin and you're cleaning it away. I really can't see why there's so much administration. I think that's what's killing the health service, I really do, because they seem to all wander around in circles all doing the same job.
(NUPE Branch secretary, Health Authority A)

In summary what we can say about this brief account of attitudes and opinions is that there are three main components to the consciousness of privatisation of this group. Firstly, there is the effect on pay and the conditions of employment which bring about the need for industrial action. Secondly, there is the factor of the effect of their actions on the community, which leads them to try to minimise the disruptive effects of their campaign. And thirdly, there is the general ideological climate towards health care and the NHS in which they are particularly inserted due to their situation and experiences. All three of these elements are combined, are competed over, and come at different times into synthesis and contradiction. In all of these elements the trade unions have a key role in, to borrow a term, their overdetermination. They affect the weighting of the elements and their relationship to one another. As a result of this, the strikers have a multiple determination of their ideas. Not only are they influenced by the "market" nature of capitalist society with its emphasis on individualism, and commodification, but they are also influenced by their economic position viz-a-viz their jobs as public sector workers.

This, when compounded with the collective values of the NHS ensures the contradictory solution we have encountered. A NUPE member at Hospital B gave a telling account of this combination when she said:

We didn't ask for more, we just want our hours back and keep contracting out. Private - it's theirs, public - its yours. And the private contractors are making big money and if there was a genuine saving in the health service you'd accept it, but you're not, you can't take that number of hours off, its unwarranted.

(NUPE member, Hospital B)

Gender oppression and political consciousness

There is one question which has not as yet been addressed and which it is important to deal with at this point. It is the question of the importance of gender. Much has been written in the last decade on the question of women's role in society. On the one hand there are those who argue that the experience of gender oppression is the fundamental one for any woman and this will mark all her experiences (Delphy, 1977; Firestone, 1979). For them, the unalterable feature of society is patriarchy and women will always be subject to the power and control of men until they combine to overthrow it. Others see the nature of society as esentially capitalist, but with strong patriarchal themes running through it (Mitchell, 1975; Barrett, 1981).

However what all share in common is the belief that it is not possible to talk of women as having the same interests and ideas as men. Thus if this is true, those women taking action against privatisation should be doing so for reasons different from those that would motivate men. Thus women's role in having principle responsibility for children would make them more aware of the social context of their dispute and make them more amenable to a campaign based around public opinion rather than industrial action, as would the fact that they are more likely to have experiences of the health service than men (Reid and Wormold, 1982) due to their perceived worse health. Also, it has been argued that women's position in the trade unions is one of sexual subordination and that their concerns are not taken seriously (Beale, 1983; Cockburn, 1983; Campbell, 1984). This could lead to a failure on behalf of the union leadership to take their dispute seriously.

In order to examine these claims two separate lines of enquiry were attempted. The first concentrated on the experiences that people had had of the NHS and how this had affected their attitude to their strike; the second attempted to establish to what degree they thought they had been treated differently because of their sex. What resulted (and this is the reason why this part was left until the end) were answers that were less than satisfactory. Questions about experiences of the NHS, produced few respondents who mentioned their own experience; some alluded to apocryphal stories about friends of friends dying before they got the operations they were on the waiting lists for. Similarly, tales were related of how disgustingly unclean the hospital now was. But in terms of any fixed level of experiences about the NHS there was little said. This may be the result of their close proximity to a dispute in the NHS in which the emphasis was on defending it. However the net result was that there was no clear evidence to support an argument that women's position in society made them more likely to be interested in defending the NHS as a service. As was pointed out above, their main motivation came from their economic circumstances not especially social ones.

The only evidence to support the importance of experience comes from the reasoning given by some strikers as to why they would not close the hospitals down. This was in the form of the "it might be my son" approach and it may suggest some connection with their position as women, but it is also true that the male trade union officials also expounded this view. It is also a quite widespread view among other strikers in essential services who explicitly do not aim to cause injury or death by their actions.

On the other linked question of the attitude of their trade union to most of those involved being women; again there was little response. What was said ranged from defence of a particular trade union official to an awareness of sexism in unions but which saw it as an extension of the leadership's traditional contempt for the rank-and-file.

> The union doesn't address itself to women even though the union is predominantly women. If you look at it in the context of how many women hold office, lay reps as well as officers, I don't think it equates with the membership; but then, the union doesn't respond to the rank and file.
> (NUPE Steward, Hospital B)

Interestingly, it was the male NUPE steward who pointed out the sexism of the hospital administration and the need to campaign over specifically women's issues. This is not to say that that the issue of gender was unimportant to the women, it was, but seemingly mainly in class terms. Thus much mention was made of the fact that the strike had taken them out of their traditional role and made them more assertive. They saw themselves very much as being in the same situation as the women in the miners" strike and made many connections with them; a fact pointing away from arguments claiming that as women they had separate interests from the male working class.

It brought us out a lot - standing up for things that I never used to before like the miners and Scargill. I'm now more militant than before.
(G & M member, Hospital B)

I'm now more aware, take more notice of things like the miners - I"m more aggressive. There's a common bond between us and them because in the end we knew it was political, we knew we were fighting the government just like them. When you are out here and you talk to these people you can relate to them.
(NUPE member, Hospital B)

I can now understand other peoples' point when they go on strike because you know what they're going through because we had never been on strike before, and we used to think about other people coming out on strike like the miners - that they're always coming out on strike. But till you've actually been on it yourself you don't realise.
(G & M member, Hospital B)

Notes

1. The methodology of the research was as follows and was developed as a response to the problems that might result from a tightly structured interview schedule. It was felt that a more effective way to discover the contradictory nature of political attitudes was to allow the subjects themselves to explain issues intheir own terms. To this end, it was decided to adopt a strategy of using semi-structured open-ended interviews. The interviews were recorded onto cassette tape recorders and the results were then transcribed into written form.

The selection of the subjects was on the basis of their involvement in some form of industrial action against privatisation / competitive tendering. This meant that to some degree those interviewed were self-selecting. This was unavoidable because opposition to the privatisation of ancillary services was in the main sporadic and geographically limited.

After an initial pilot study the following eight questions general themes were developed to be used in interviews with ancillary workers.
1. Why were they taking industrial action? / Why had they taken industrial action?
2. What did they see as the issues involved in their action?
3. Why has privatisation come about and what does it represent?
4. What limits would they put on their action and why?

5. What did they feel about private medicine and private health insurance?

6. How did they conceive of the NHS and how did they envisage it could be improved?

7. What experiences did they have of the NHS themselves?

8. What effect did the fact that they were women have on their treatment by the union?

Questions put to the trade union officials / campaign co- ordinators followed the same pattern except for the exclusion of the last two questions and the inclusion of two new questions. These were on the role of public opinion and what strategy they saw as having most chance of success. These questions were added for obvious reasons which are discussed in the main text.

The written data was analysed by a process of identifying the main themes in each interview and building up a composite picture of the responses to them. This is described in chapters Five, Six and Seven. In this way, what could be described as an "ideal type" was constructed. This process is described in Bulmer (1975, pp 171-172) where he emphasizes its role as a "heuristic device" - rather than as a Weberian methodological principle. Because it is its role as a tool aiding interpretation that is foremost, it is unnecessary, therefore, to justify its "truthfulness" (as against its "falsity'"), rather what is important is its "fruitfulness" in terms of aiding research.

What also needs to be emphasised is that for most interviewees the questions were merely prompts for them to articulate their own ideas. Consequently, many "answers" did not correspond to the "questions". Interviewees touched upon many themes before they are mentioned as a topic of discussion. Far from being an obstacle to study, this resulted in making it easier to construct a composite picture of the opinions of the group.

5 Ideology and the privatisation of NHS ancillary services: The view from the leadership

The previous chapter examined the attitudes towards privatisation taken by striking ancillary workers. What started as a simple strike in response to new working conditions became a struggle between conflicting social values and ideas about health. Awareness of this struggle also affected ancillary workers' ability to successfully conclude their dispute. Finally, it was also asserted that even in their adoption of one side of this value divide, an absolute dichotomy was not created. In other words their value systems as they related to the public / private health care split were of a partial nature.

The reader is reminded of this at this point because of the important role that the interviewees' trade union officials had in influencing the conduct and direction of their disputes. In line with the general approach of this work, what I shall be arguing is that the emphasis put on the ideological struggle by the strikers themselves was partially the consequence of the attitude towards privatisation of the trade unions as mediated through their officials.

It could be argued that this emphasis on the ideological could only have beneficial effects for the strikers in that it extended the weapons available to them. However, when viewed as an alternative to using industrial action (as the trade union leaders often did) it could only lead to the stagnation and ultimate failure of the anti-privatisation struggles. This is important for this study because it reflects the essential difference in approach of those giving priority to winning hegemony at, effectively, a intellectual level over those adopting a more traditional stance, and as such it relates to the overall project of this study.

The existence of many ideas not in accordance with the notion of the welfare state by these privatised workers points to a considerable failure of the counter-hegemonic model. If those that are directly affected by privatisation cannot be wholly won over, then who can. Of course it would be naive to believe that a consistent industrial struggle would have done any better, but, if conducted in such a way as to connect the industrial struggle with politics it might have produced a more thorough going position on the part of the rank-and-file than that which was produced. This could have been achieved by giving them the feeling that they had the ability to do more than just defend what was in the process of being taken away from them. Their involvement in such practical activity would have potentially allowed them to universalize their experience in much the same way that the women strikers at Hospital B saw the "point of view" of other strikers.

This chapter then, is concerned with examining the views of Trade union officials towards privatisation. Though, only a small number of full-time officials and strike co-ordinators were interviewed (thus inviting the criticism of the sample not providing sufficient evidence to be able to generalise from), the very fact that they displayed a considerable degree of consensus over a number of important issues suggests that a large amount of agreement does exist among this layer of officialdom. On top of this can be added the correspondence of their views with the health service unions' published views. Also, and this is again an important factor, those interviewed had strong connections with the ancillary workers interviewed earlier in that they were the officers responsible for organising them[1]. A strong case can be made not only for the coherence of their views, but also for the effect their opinions had further down the hierarchy.

What needs to be established from the outset, is that it was not the case that there was an immediate articulation of the anti-privatisation strategy as counter-hegemonic by any of the officials. Rather, there was the slow development of this strategy out of the general approach to privatisation adopted by them. Privatisation was seen differently by the officials because they started from a different relationship with it, the starting point of the ancillary towards privatisation was in essence economic, while that of the of the officials was political. This can be clearly seen in way privatisation is described:

Privatisation is totally ideological - they want to see the NHS and all public institutions broken up and they want to see private industry running them rather than the NHS. So there's a totally ideological reason for it - they're committed to private enterprise, totally committed to destroying the basis of the health service and other public bodies. So the introduction of private tendering and private contractors is a step in that direction and the other party part of that, which is another factor in my opinion, is that they don't like the fact that the NHS does have strong trade union organisation within it, and the majority of the staff, particularly manual workers, are organised into trade unions and are prepared to complain about their wages and conditions - the government doesn't like that, and so it also wants to break the power of the trade unions and one way of doing that is to privatise and either use that as a weapon to reduce trade union power by frightening workers into accepting reductions in wages and conditions, or, directly to bring private firms that don't recognise trade unions in order to break the power of collective bargaining. So from every angle I see the attack as being a totally ideological one upon both the basis of the welfare state and upon trade union organisation.

(Official, Health Authority A)

As can be seen here, two aspects are apparent (and these are similar to the attitudes of other officials) - that privatisation represents a political threat to both the welfare state and to the unions / workers. Already, the threat to the welfare state is as important as the effects on the people the official is supposed to represent.

Even when the full time officials attribute privatisation to the pressure to reduce public expenditure this factor is present:

Financially the government is committed to reducing state expenditure. They claim they see state expenditure as a burden on profit-making industries and therefore they want to reduce state expenditure. So there again that's in line with their political beliefs in terms of running capitalism. From the point of view from which they see running capitalism they want to reduce public expenditure and so the additional factor is that they can reduce public expenditure by privatising it. They believe by competitive tendering which results in staff agreeing to worse conditions and wages for themselves and that reduces costs and staffing. Or by bringing private firms that are going to achieve the same objective and are not really concerned about the end product, about

whether it works well or whether its carrying out the service. They're just concerned with the saving of money full stop.
(Official, Health Authority A)

From the above two statements it can be seen that what started out as the union's principle point of entry into the whole issue of privatisation, the effect that it had on its members had quickly, if not immediately, become a constitutive element of a wider political question. For the official the economic and the political sides to privatisation were inextricably linked. For them it was only a matter of time before this became apparent to the rank-and-file, and presumably, as politics is more important than economics, it would be the political motivation that would become uppermost in their minds. Of course, it is not unusual for union leaders to be more politicised than their members, but what is unusual is these officials' ability to make the politics the integral element of trade union activity. Even the NUM only campaigned over pay rates in their disputes of the 1970s. And even though it brought up many other issues, the 1984-85 miners' strike was over job losses and not the moral nature of the coal industry (though some thought it should have been). Talking of the relationship between the different motivations, the same official went on to say:

> I think the two (politics and economics) are related to one another. I think that its very difficult to divorce economic and political factors and I think the two are tied to each other, and one to a very large extent determines the other, but I think that many of the workers that took strike action against privatisation, did so initially on the grounds that they were concerned that they would be out of a job - because the women at Hospital A came out when it was recommended that they go to private contractors, so they were fighting for their jobs, but in the course of that, and even at the time they made their decision they were also saying that we don't want to see this hospital going into the ground: we've worked in it for a number of years, fifteen years, in the case of some of them, twenty years, we know patients, we like our work, we don't want to see all that destroyed which is what a private contractor will do if they come in with considerably less staff. So that was tied up with it as well. So there obviously was self-motivation in a sense, people don't want to lose their jobs and they need a job because that money is important, its not pin money in the way its been portrayed, its an important part of the family income, a lot of them single parents and widows and

100

people relying on that income; but tied up with that you've got political factors as well and of course as the dispute and the political arguments develop, those political factors become more and more important because they saw what was taking place, what was happening.

(Official, Health Authority A)

In this way the whole issue of privatisation's effect on medical care and health provision came to the fore because here the two issues of staffing and health policy can be combined. Privatisation makes hospitals dirtier and reduces health care by reducing the number of staff. As one NUPE leaflet put it: "contract cleaning firms are knocking at the door, wherever they've come in, care's gone out the window". This was reflected in the view of an official who, when asked whether the ideal of public health had much effect on the way members viewed privatisation, replied:

Perhaps not in the same sense as the union as such, I think they find it in their own work being affected ... If you take the domestics, a lot of them enjoy the job because there's a lot of personal contact with the patients and other people in the hospital and so it is done on very much of a community basis the nursing staff are very hard-pressed and so the domestic staff take on additional duties they don't get paid for. Privatisation doesn't take this into account - it isn't quantified, that sort of job satisfaction and contact. It results in a loss in patient care and a reducing down of the caring aspect of the service, which in turn, and this is the argument, and obviously this is the government's plan, they're turning it into a second rate service that isn't providing the level of care we need.

(Official, Health Authority C)

That these views were consensual and in harmony with the union's general approach can be seen by a brief look at the materials used by NUPE in their campaign against privatisation. These include:

* A set of three educational broadsheets:

"Broadsheet 1 sets NHS privatisation in the context of the government's wider strategy of transferring public industries and services over to private hands. It points out the flaws in the government's argument for contracting out".

"Broadsheet 2 looks at common misunderstandings about the threat of contractors such as "I don't know what all the fuss is about, working for contractors will be no different to working for the NHS". This broadsheet answers directly this and other questions providing useful information for activists".

"Broadsheet 3 examines how the union can successfully resist privatisation by the combined use of trade union action and community support".

* Posters and leaflets on the following topics:

NUPE says "Stop the Cuts"
NUPE says "Save the Health Service"
NUPE Health warning : "No Private Con tricks Here!"
NUPE Health warning : "Contractors Put Profit Before People" NUPE Health warning : "Public it's Yours Private it's Theirs" Hands Off the NHS Private Contractors Keep Out
NUPE says "Care not Profit in the NHS"

* Leaflets

Private Contractors Failures in the NHS
Who Cares? We Do! Health Service Under Attack No Private Contricks Here
Contractors Put Profits Before People
Public It's Yours Private It's Theirs

Alongside this a number videos were also produced (Safe in our hands, Griffiths Report on the NHS) all containing roughly the same message - that privatisation is a double attack, on both the staff and on the NHS itself.

While the emphasis of any trade unions work has got to be its own membership, the effect of highlighting the "attack on the NHS"; while motivated by attempts to defend them, leads logically to an emphasis on the views of the General Public. In this way it can be seen how the nature of the NHS ancillary's job led to the adoption of a strategy of struggle at the level of public opinion. Much of the union's activity was centred around trying to gain their support. The slogans on posters designed by NUPE were as much chosen for their impact on the public as they were on their ability to mobilise their members. This is as true of the leaflets produced as it is of the posters. The themes of the leaflets shown above were predominantly about the effect on services not on conditions.

As I have been arguing, this was not accidental. By sleight of hand or otherwise, the emphasis of the unions anti-privatisation struggle was on the public, and to win their support it was necessary to address their interests directly. The text of a local leaflet shows how this was done:

SAVING MONEY?

"When you've worked as a domestic on the wards for a few years, you get to know which patients are anxious or frightened. Working around their beds, serving them their meals, making them a hot drink - you soon establish a relationship with them. Gradually you can reassure them and build up their confidence - especially the old ones. Its all part of getting well.

Or was.

Contract cleaning firms are knocking at the door. Wherever they've come in, care's gone out the window.

Caring's our life. We know we're needed. And right now we know we need your support."

SAVE THE NHS

This leaflet was put out as part of the Health Focus Week (22nd - 26th April 1985) organised by all the health service unions. This again showed the dominant strategy behind the health service unions' approach. Health Focus Week was not about organising a week of industrial action against privatisation, rather it was designed as a propaganda exercise. Rodney Bickerstaffe writing of the effects of privatisation in a special health focus edition of the NUPE Standard wrote:

> NUPE urges all NHS staff to use Health Focus Week from April 22-26 as an opportunity to reach out beyond their own workplaces and alert our communities about the poison of Thatcherism.
>
> We must strengthen our own organisation both inside and outside

the workplace. It is vital that staff at the sharp end of Tory cuts and privatisation plans are not left to fight alone.

Don't let Thatcher break up the health care team. Together we can defend our jobs and the health of ordinary people. It is time to step up the action.

The union's position on privatisation as adopted at the 1984 annual conference ran along similar lines:

Conference recognises that privatisation is part of a political strategy which aims to reduce and eliminate services and institutions established over the last forty years for the benefit of working people. Therefore we believe that although privatisation is being introduced by individual councils and health authorities it will only be beaten as a strategy at national level. Conference believes that fighting individual employers in isolated struggles is no substitutes for a campaign against the policies of a government and also recognises that the same policies are designed to replace "service" with "profit" as the motive in the operation of key publicly controlled industries such as gas, electricity and telephones.

Conference calls upon the executive council to:
a)Co-Ordinate a vigorous campaign at national and local levels to educate the public about the vital importance of public services and the need to defend them in the face of Tory cuts and privatisation.
b)Pursue within the TUC and for other appropriate channels links with all unions in the public sector resisting privatisation (eg. telecom and GPO unions, NUM, civil service unions) to co-ordinate action and establish a joint publicity campaign to combat the anti public sector policies and propaganda emanating from the government and the media respectively.
c)Co-Ordinate and publicise widely all fights against privatisation and mount an effective national campaign including national days of action national demonstrations, etc.
d)Give maximum support to all members opposing the use of contractors.

It is clear then that as far as the full-time leadership of the union were concerned the question of privatisation was one of competing political ideologies and social value systems. Privatisation has its importance as a key way of undermining the welfare state and its ethos of "service" rather than "profit". To quote the National Education Officer of NUPE:

Privatisation in the NHS was designed by this government to try and break into the NHS and put back the profit motive into Medicine in this country. Now, the government will never admit that they will say - it has all to do with value for money, efficiency etc. That's all verbal diarrhoea...as far as the government is concerned what it has done is to reintroduce, for the first time since 1948, the profit motive.

The concern they have for their members quickly became a more general concern for the state of public welfare, a concern that they wished to transmit to the population at large and in turn involve them in its defence. This affected the way in which they perceived tactical questions over how privatisation was to be opposed. It will be noticed how the conference resolution quoted earlier devoted very little attention to opposing privatisation through industrial means. On the contrary it seemed to counterpose this strategy to one where education and alliance building were primary. It explicitly says that "isolated struggles" are no substitute for a "strategy at a national level".

What did this national strategy actually mean in practice. Concretely, the resolution stated that the government should be pressurised by MP's of all parties to bring about the immediate restoration of legislation to ensure fair wages and conditions for all workers, be they publicly or privately employed. This being a step to getting a Labour government to renationalise all privatised sectors of the economy.

It was this strategy that predominated, even in the light of the 1983 conference decision to organise "a national campaign of industrial action" against privatisation and its reiteration in support of the Hospital B strikers in 1984. Even though the union was firmly resolved "to take national industrial action to determine a victorious outcome", it is not this strategy that motivated the union.

How then did this understanding influence the conduct of the union in actual circumstances of privatisation? The cases before us are of three different outcomes to the implementation of privatisation. At Hospital B the resistance was immediate and total leading to a strike that continued for over eighteen months. In Health authority A the result was the same at first with a strike by ancillary workers lasting a few days but which ultimately went down to defeat. At Hospital C, an initial hostility to privatisation resulted in a campaign but no strike action. The reasons for the, at one level at least, positive response at Hospital B are probably explicable in terms of the support structure offered by the local support organisation which was outside the official structure of NUPE. This will be returned to later as it helps to highlight the nature of NUPE's position. But the examples of Health Authority A and Hospital C are probably more interesting in that here the campaigns failed. The two full-time officials involved regarded the failure of these and other similar disputes as deriving from a lack of confidence of those under threat. This is even more suprising when the political differences that exist between them are taken into account, for despite their intentions they come to conclusions which belie their advocacy of industrial action.

> There is certainly a gap between people's hatred of privatisation and what's happening to them, and translating that into taking industrial action to achieve objectives, and I think the main reason is that the unions themselves don't have confidence in their own ability to defeat their employer. They rightly see that the government is responsible and that they are to achieve their objective they've got to bring down the government. There's a sense in which what they're saying is absolutely right,... I don't think this myself but there can be a lack of confidence among workers themselves about their ability to fight. They don't see that they've got some strength and some ability and they don't see what impact their dispute would have if they were to fight within their locality. Having said that, I think that the trade union leadership bears some responsibility because I don't believe that they have started to develop their confidence enough. I think that many of the leaders have been giving signals - that we can't defeat the employers and we're not going to get anywhere and if they start to say things like that in public, and there have been plenty of examples of those types of things being said in public, then that only goes back to reinforce the mood that exists at the bottom; that we can't win and that reinforces the view of the people at the top that we can't win either, and so we all disappear up our arses doing nothing: and I think in general terms that is what has happened over the past few years and it boils down to a very poor lead that has been given from top trade union leaders.
>
> (Official, Health Authority A)

At Hospital C:

> I think they realised it wasn't down to them entirely in the sense that industrial action, if they were going to take any further action

it was going to be token action..... I think they saw once the contractors were there, if they were going to stay on the picket line they would be there a long time, they had seen so many of their colleagues beaten and although there was a lot of sympathy and people got guilty and such and took part in the demonstrations, there wasn't this mass reaction against privatisation and that contributed a lot to it.

(Official, Health Authority C)

Whilst politically very different these two officials identified the lack of confidence that their members had in winning against privatisation as a major problem. This is further substantiated by the account of the dispute put up at Hospital C:

I think they tended to, as people tend to do, sit and wait and see what happens when the contract arrived then the evils we had been warning them about, that was the time they reacted. They felt they had been cheated... its the way they handle it (the health authority) at shop floor level, they say "well don't get involved in any nonsense and we might keep the service in-house and everything will be alright here".

Everything you try to get off the ground you've got the whole management force trying to squash you - very difficult in this part of the world to get that early reaction, and in fact we really didn't get any reaction until what we'd been saying had taken off. Initially there was a meeting out there, the contractors turned up and gave a list of the appalling conditions they were prepared to offer everyone. They all got up and walked out and rang up my self and said they wanted a meeting over there and from there it took off.

I think initially they felt cheated that they had been lied to by the health authority ... and in all directions, and then as the campaign developed to keep them out, then I think it moved into another phase of where they were aware of how the service was going to be affected because they then started to look at ways of contacting others. In the final analysis when the contract in, we were prepared to move into an adequate bargaining position and have them all out on strike there. But, unlike Hospital B and Addenbrookes they wanted to throw in the towel - the furthest they could get away from the hospital the better they didn't want any more to do with it - they didn't want to stand on a picket line for a year to fight for it.

(Official, Health Authority C)

Crucial then, became the support of groups outside of the hospitals to make up for this deficiency, and here the argument comes full circle, putting the emphasis on the outside world. This is not to suggest however, that there was a neat equation between this and seeking to win public opinion, it can also mean an extension of industrial struggle to these other groups. Nevertheless, it does mean moving away from a strategy focused upon health service industrial action, to one where this is just a component. This point comes over from the Health Authority official when discussing whether closing one hospital down completely would lead to success:

I think that's highly unlikely, I see the need for health service workers to link up with private industry for instance, and we saw a glimmer of that in the 1979 dispute, even if only on a token basis with groups like in the mining industry and in private factories striking in solidarity with the health service workers. And I see that type of pressure as being the way we're actually going to succeed, rather than saying we'll kill off all patients in Dartford or something.

(Official, Health Authority A)

Or another view:

My view is that we have got to fight privatisation, whenever we can, whatever way we can, and mobilise those forces that will stand and fight privatisation, involve all the groups we can where in-house tenders have been won. Because my belief is that there is only one solution - that's a political solution - I don't think there's an industrial solution to it. It has to be decided, I believe, by an incoming Labour Government who would be committed to kicking privatisation out of the health service and it will be an easier job to do if the damage is minimised - we talk of irreversible socialism - it's irreversible capitalism. My fear is that the next Labour government won't have this high on its list of priorities. But that actually seems to be the best defence - to actually come up with some wonderful blueprint, some plan by industrial means, sort of raise the level of awareness, mobilise all the forces that you need to do it - overturn privatisation. I think its a bit of a long shot.

(Official, Health Authority A)

What this did then, in the context of there being few groups ready to add their muscle to the anti-privatisation cause, was to reinforce the importance of opposing privatisation on a moral or community basis. The struggle was one in which there were two competing systems of health care; one market based, the other need based, and it was this struggle that became the motivating principle of the activities against privatisation. So much so, that hospital workers who originally came out and took action over the effects of privatisation on their livelihoods were encouraged to see their struggle in these ideological terms. Thus in terms of the evidence presented above, most ancillaries who had taken action over privatisation have echoed the belief that what was occurring was a dismantling of the nationalised public health system in Britain by the Government. At the same time, because these individuals still exist in a world of market relationships, they have accepted the need and existence of a private health system outside of the NHS. This is an important difference with the union position as represented by the officials. For the officials operate outside the constraints of the economic world, for them opinions and attitudes have to be consistent and allow for no contradiction.

> My own view is that we shouldn't allow the private sector to exist at all, my own view is that a Labour Government should legislate against any private practice in the health service at all, that you shouldn't allow private health service at all, that you shouldn't allow private hospitals and you shouldn't allow private health, full stop. Not only inside the national health service but outside as well, it should be prohibited.
>
> (Official, Health Authority A)

For this official the explanation of this position resides in the role played by the NHS in creating the conditions for existence of the private sector.

> Well there's a number of things you can go into that are suggested by the argument; the first is that if you have a private health care alternative to the NHS, within certainly the system you have now, that inevitably means you have a two tier system and those that can afford things will get better things, but that system is still dependent on the National Health Service, the majority of nurses

and the majority of doctors are trained at public expense through publicly funded institutions and through the NHS. The majority of the development of the equipment of the NHS is carried out through the health service. The major expenditure on major equipment only the NHS can afford and inevitably what happens is, and this is what is happening today even if we excluded private care within the NHS. Private care outside the health service is dependent on the NHS for a supply of trained staff, for equipment that has been used and all the rest of it. And so inevitably the private sector couldn't exist without the public sector. So I have my views that would simply say that these things aren't allowed and I'd extend it further, I don't think we should have private education, I think all private schools should be banned too.

(Official, Health Authority A)

What is interesting about this view is that it contains nearly all the same elements of antagonism to private health that the rank and file have articulated, except for one important difference, namely that they still recognise the right of individuals to buy for themselves private health care as long as it was totally separate from the health service. For the official the argument needs to be consistent if it is to function effectively as an ideology and here an important dimension of this study becomes apparent, namely that for the official's ideology plays a much more important motivating role than for the rank and file. Significantly, it feeds into an approach that attaches more importance to ideological struggle. This becomes intensified in the circumstances of privatisation, not just because of its overt political nature but also because of the obvious lack of success in combating competitive tendering in purely trade union terms. As the industrial struggle falters or becomes bogged down in long drawn out disputes, so the officials either see the solution as lying with an incoming Labour Government or with the present government creating such a wave of discontent that a generalised industrial struggle will break out, politicising its participants and bringing about a general election.

Hence the constant reference of the group to disputes such as Hospital B's acting as a "conscience" on other union members and the public in general (although of course, the precise role that this conscience plays is different depending on the political perspective of the individual articulating it):

Hospital B and Addenbrookes... dare I say this, its almost blasphemy, by standing on a picket line for a year or something

110

they are a sort of conscience for privatisation, but in industrial terms of whether you're actually achieving anything by your action is what I think is the real interpretation of industrial action - you withdraw your labour for the sake of achieving an end because you have then stopped the means of production or service, then I think clearly then Addenbrookes and Hospital B are not doing that."

(Official, Health Authority C)

Addenbrookes and Hospital B have acted like a conscience for everybody else, everybody is thinking in the back of their minds really "if we were out there with them as well, then perhaps we could defeat privatisation" and that's in the back of peoples' minds and the more these disputes continue to fight the more in the back of someones' mind will be "only if we had done it as well".

(Official, Health Authority A)

The attitudes of the rank and file did not mirror those of their officials, their motivation stems far more from their circumstances than from ideological imperatives. They were not inclined to see disputes over privatisation as beacons, rather they simply wished to win them. If they felt they were unlikely to do so they would stop acting. At Hospital B the reason the dispute entered its second year was more to do with securing better industrial tribunal compensation than with acting out any vanguard role. Nevertheless they did stress their predicament in the hope of getting solidarity action from other hospitals, but essentially as a means of winning their own dispute.

That the union officials viewed the anti-privatisation campaign as essentially an ideological dispute can be gleaned from the views of the strike workers at the support group for Hospital B. These individuals, though full-time officials (they were funded by the metropolitan council and for a time by the union itself), had as their main concern the organisation and success of the Hospital B dispute rather than the administration of a trade union. As a result of trying to pursue this aim they became highly critical of the way the union viewed the dispute and the whole issue of privatisation. This animosity became mutual when, during the middle of the dispute, the union withdrew its funding of the strike worker that they paid for.

In terms of setting the scene it is also important to be aware that the original involvement of the support group in the dispute was because a trade union support group also involved a number of other NUPE members. These had gone forward to the strikers to offer their support as trade unionists and the specific involvement of the strike support group as an organisation stemmed from this. In the early stages of the dispute the union welcomed this support, even going so far as to fund a strike worker. One support group worker described the early days in the following terms:

> The strike had taken on a greater magnitude, gained a lot of publicity. People used to dealing with the press had got the story over, and we'd used it very much in that way. NUPE was very much in support of the dispute in the early days. GMBATU had a much lower profile because it had a minority of members taking part.
>
> (Support group worker, Hospital B)

At the beginning the dispute attracted a lot of attention and was popular with the union leadership. This situation soon changed when instead of burning out, the strike kept going and the strikers started to demand effective solidarity in the form of a national campaign of industrial action:

> ...continually the call being made to our union was - we need a strategy to fight privatisation, we need to combine our energies to fight privatisation. The ideal of trade unionism is that you don't fight alone, that you pull in people around you and use all your resources as well as possible. And this simply isn't happening as far as I know - there isn't, even now, a strategy or programme to look at privatisation and fight privatisation.
>
> (Support group worker, Hospital B)

Because of this failure on the part of the union, the support group workers became more and more critical of a strategy based on public opinion as the only way forward. This is not to say that they saw no role for the mobilisation of public opinion, but that it was of secondary importance:

> It is very easy for them to appeal to what is the most common interest - which is a good health service. But you can have a good service in South Africa on slave wages. A trade union leaders responsibility is to his members and that's very much how trade unionists see it. If they are going to carry out this campaign or policy of raising the health issues - which are an advantage - then it should be done in the same way as we did it; with a separate

112

organisation representing that interest
(Support group worker, Hospital B)

For the support group workers the pursuit of a strategy geared to winning public opinion had the danger of turning unions into what one of them called "unions of rhetoric", where they ignored the nitty-gritty issues of pay and industrial relations in favour of an emphasis on "the next Labour government". For them, this trend was exemplified by the then NUPE General Secretary Rodney Bickerstaffe's description of the Hospital B Dispute as "Our Cortonwood". However, as they point out; for the NUM the closure of Cortonwood was the signal for an all-out strike, for NUPE it was the signal for increased platitudes. Thus, they concluded:

> There is an industrial solution, they've got seats - Bickerstaffe sits on the TUC - unions are powerful. If there isn't [an industrial solution] why have "no strike deals". They will look for any other solution - apart from involving their members in action.
> (Support group worker, Hospital B)

> The health unions are powerful enough to win. You've got to look at the reasons why they haven't. If that conference resolution had been taken up and built upon, like it should have been and you got hospital workers out on strike and you are preventing hospitals from working, then you're powerful enough. But if you've got officials going about and saying to people, as they did in the strike - you take action and we can't guarantee your jobs, then its no wonder you fail.
> (Support group worker, Hospital B)

This brings the discussion back to the question of the interests of the patients against those of the strikers. In many ways this is the crucial question. For in favouring one group over another, one must choose one's overall strategy: industrial or ideological. For the support group workers the choice was simple:

> I turned away items because I was there on a picket line, I was there because of the jobs - the interests of the members. And once you carry out this "the health issue", then you're taking responsibility for that area - which is not the remit of union officials. You don't get Arthur Scargill talking about the quality of coal or whatever. That's not his concern. Once they jump on that

113

bandwagon its a downhill trip.
(Support group worker, Hospital B)

These views, then, coming as they do from a group outside of our simple dichotomy, put into relief the strategy being pursued by the union hierarchy and probably account for some of the confusion of the Hospital B strikers who found them selves being pulled in two directions at the same time. Their emphasis on industrial struggle did not exclude the raising of the more general issues, indeed, the support group's work in gaining the support of the community put the national union to shame. But, it was a subordinate campaign and in the differing circumstances of, say, the union's wholehearted support for a campaign of national industrial action, it could have been used to break down divisions between different groups of workers by linking them to a common cause and by asking them to deliver solidarity action, politicising them. However, in the circumstances of tokenistic action designed to serve as an "example" of the effect of Tory policies, it had the result of demoralising the union rank-and-file by leaving them isolated as well as leaving the vast majority of people as passive observers.

What has been presented is a practical demonstration of the development of trade union struggle as counter-hegemonic alliance building. A strategy which, as has been pointed out before, takes much of its justification from the nature of the work that its members do. It is a strategy that resulted from combining the traditional reticence of the trade union hierarchy for industrial action with the influence of "New Revisionist" theory. It is also a strategy that failed. It was not effective in countering the development of privatisation; neither did it swing public opinion massively in favour of socialism, or what for them is the same thing, electoral support for the Labour Party. As I will proceed to argue, this was inevitable given their detachment of ideology and politics from processes of practical political activity at the economic level. The solution, if that is the right word, to their attempts to create a hegemonic politics can only be realised by the close linking of economic issues with those of a political nature. This connection can only occur if it is based on the the practical activity of the workers themselves. Ultimately, this must also involve the politicisation and generalisation, and on occasion, the conscious direction of struggles by organisations of the most politically advanced sections of the working class; that is by socialist parties.

114

Notes

1. They were: the full-time official responsible for Health Authority A, the full-time official responsible for Health Authority C, and the full-time workers in Hospital B working to coordinate the Hospital B dispute.

6 Counter-hegemonic struggle and the limitations of political consciousness

What then can be said about the ideas and opinions held by the group of ancillary workers studied? And more importantly, what have been the effects on them of the trade unions' counter-hegemonic strategy? Before we can answer these questions we must first be aware that opinions and ideologies are not things that arise spontaneously out of social intercourse, but rather are contested, fought over, and generally exist in a state of constant dispute. A political consciousness is not formed at any one point in time and neither does it remain unchanged by the situations it finds itself in.

As has been indicated before, what we have occurring in the circumstances of privatisation are a number of different struggles over different ideological terrains. At its most simplistic it is the struggle of the trade unions to get their members to oppose the implementation of privatisation. This must, of necessity, involve an appeal to their economic interests. At its most complicated, however, it involves a clash between competing conceptions of how the world should be ordered; on the basis of the dictates of the market or on the basis of social need? In between these two polarities there are a whole series of other conflicts; between ideological and industrial methods of conducting the dispute; over who runs the dispute - the leadership or the strikers themselves; even conflicts over strategy - whether or not to keep the picket-lines going.

The purpose of assessing these conflicts is to show how the pursuit of an ideological campaign by the unions is incapable of even fully winning over a group so centrally involved in the issue, let alone those more distanced from the issue. The argument that will be presented is that in basing themselves so firmly on the winning of an ideological victory, the promoters of counter-hegemonic politics in the trade unions failed to take account of the tremendous power that capitalist social relations exert in the creation of opinion. This is because such relations are rooted firmly in the every-day existence of all individuals. Because of this, counter-hegemonists can only have at best a superficial impact on the consciousness of any group of those individuals.[1]

Consequently, it must be apparent that these ideological contests, which are at the heart of the counter-hegemonists position, are not between evenly matched rivals. Instead, the ideas which the unions and socialists have to contest have the advantage of being deeply rooted in the very structure of capitalist social formations. The idea of the market, for example, penetrates into every aspect of life, starting with the need for the worker to sell his/her labour for a "fair" price and moving up to the "right" of individuals to "purchase" any commodity they may require, such as health care or even sex. In this way, there is a contestation of ideas going on at every level of society, one which is loaded in favour of the interests of the dominant classes. This, however, does not mean that those in the subordinate classes are completely devoid of resources to counter this influence. Working class experiences, although moulded by hegemonic forces, cannot totally be integrated into a "grey" monolithic dominant ideology; rather, the dominant accounts of their situations which pervade society are negotiated by the members of the subordinate classes into new, if often partial, ideological forms. These forms are often replicas of the dominant culture but they also exhibit contradictory elements as well. For all its limitations trade unionism could not have come into existence without such a process occurring. It is this notion of ideological transformation that provides the key to the understanding of the ideas of the NHS ancillaries in this study.

What occurred was that the NHS ancillaries, motivated by a desire to preserve their conditions of employment became involved in a struggle that is primarily ideological. They adopted positions through expediency and through the arguments making sense to them. The influence of just pure ideology is not enough to overcome the basic ideas of any society. As we have pointed out above, these have their foundation in capitalist relations of production. This is the origin of the particular contradictions that we have seen.

The question of the abolition of private medicine illustrates this by

117

pointing to a divergence between the thought of the officials and that of the membership. For while the rank-and-file rejected profit as the basis for care within the health service they also accepted the existence and the right to have private health care outside of the NHS. The officials, on the other hand, accepted no such right. This divergence goes further when the institutional make-up of the NHS is examined, especially in the light of the 1945 Labour election victory and the creation of the welfare state. For an official:

> The 1945 creation was about a number of things, first of all a landslide victory for Labour at that time, a determination by the troops coming back from fighting that they didn't want to see what happened in the 30s happen again, a determination that they wanted to build something better which got Labour returned on a landslide victory on a programme that was very radical at the time - and meant a number of advances particularly the establishment of the NHS but even so I would say it was a compromise with various things for instance the ability to continue private practice for instance being embodied into the way in which the health service was set up. But I think the problem with the state industries, and I include the NHS in that, is the way it was set up and managed - it was still seen as management from the top, some bureaucrats appointed through the state machinery rather than management from the bottom by the workers themselves or involving workers and trade unions and the people who actually work and benefit from the service and I think thats been the problem in the NHS, the Coal Board, the British Steel industry, electricity industry, the water industry, all the public services suffer from the same problem.
>
> (Official, Health Authority A)

For the rank-and-file the nature of the NHS and its creation is not so clear. There is a constant invocation of the principles under which it was founded, as well as continual reference to the fact that it was an achievement that was admired throughout the world. However, there is also a belief that it is not run as efficiently as it could be and that it is misused:

> There's a lot to be desired in the national health, the way it's run definitely, someone ought to get there and sort it out. Its a pity old Bevan died really. He knew what we wanted, but they all misused it in the end, didn't they? I don't think he'd be very happy

118

with what it is now.

(G&M member, Hospital B)

The NHS should be run by hospital administrators not outsiders.

(NUPE member, Health Authority A)

When questioned about how they would like to see the NHS develop all answers were about the allocation of resources and none about the potential control that they could exercise over it. It could be that in directing the emphasis of the campaign on to the question of health it encouraged the rank-and-file to think of themselves as consumers rather than as producers and in this way ensured that the question of control did not enter into the debate. It is also true that from the very inception of the NHS the question of workers' control has never really figured, possibly showing a lack of interest on all sides to the idea.

What is possibly of more importance to this discrepancy of views is the role played by the individual ancillary worker as, to borrow Poulantzas' term, a "juridico-political individual" (Poulantzas, 1975), though this importance is not immediately apparent. What is under discussion here, is that according to democratic theory an individual's participation in the structure of a society provides to that individual certain rights and obligations. This is understood by most people implicitly, if not explicitly, eg. the vote, taxation etc. Privatisation by seemingly removing free access to health care is seen by the ancillary workers as going against those rights.

I don't think you should have to pay private you're already paying your contributions, some people take a lot out of the health service and some don't never need it, that's fortunate for them in one way because they're healthy. But you pay your stamps. I think it's a disgusting situation for the very poor, its not a fair system.

(NUPE member, Hospital B)

I thought this is what you paid your stamp for, national health and all that, but she's doing away with it, privatising everything, so you're going to end up paying to go into hospital and have anything done, we couldn't afford to do that.

(G&M member, Hospital B)

As a result of the form taken by this argument an awareness is created of one of the first counteracting tendencies existing at the ideological

119

level to the creation of a homogeneous anti-market welfare ideology. By constituting all individuals as component units in an organic whole, the theory precludes a understanding of the politics and interests that lie behind the artificial unity that it creates. In understanding this process it is useful to look at Marx's treatment of Hegel in his two essays "On the Jewish Question" and "A Contribution to the Critique of Hegel's Philosophy of Right".

Hegel in his work on the state makes a distinction between civil society where private interests conflict and the state which operates in the general interest. Colletti (1975) describes it in this way:

> In "civil society" - which for Hegel as for Adam Smith and Ricardo was a "market-society" of producers - individuals are divided from and independent of one another. Under such conditions just as each person is independent of all others, so does the real nexus of mutual dependence (the bond of social unity) become in turn independent of all individuals. This common interest or "universal" interest renders itself independent of all the interested parties and assumes a separate existence: and such social unity established in separation from its members is, precisely, the hypostatized modern state.
>
> (Colletti, 1975 pp.256-257)

Walton (1983) points out, that what is primary for Hegel is civil society and its diverse interests, consequently, the state can be conceived of as nothing other than an elaborate institutional mechanism for coordinating those interests. He writes:

> On this view, the public interest is what is necessary for the coordination of private interests. Further, on this view, the role of the state is that of securing private interests in so far as it enforces the public interest. This is what Hegel calls the state "based on need", the state which is the means to securing private interests.
>
> (Walton, 1983, p260)

For Hegel the dialectic between the individual interest and the public interest is mediated by what he describes as ethical life. Ethical life for Hegel consisted of the complex of shared norms and values that derive from the common, historically nurtured experience of people living together in a shared culture. Through the particular actions and agency of individuals there develops a universal of ethical life. This provides the basis for a collective concern about the health and welfare of all sections of the community and a corresponding commitment to state activity.

This commitment derives from a rejection of private charity and alms giving as a means of helping the poor. Helping the poor cannot be left to "private sympathy" and the "charitable disposition" of particular individuals. On the contrary, it is the obligation of the community as whole, acting throught the state, to provide for the needs of those afflicted by the consequences of economic crisis. The remedying of poverty is thus a "universal" as opposed to a "particular" activity, and as such it expresses the ethical life of the community. Modern ethical life embodies generally shared norms and values governing relations between individuals and groups: it embraces shared principles of justice and reasonable equality, and these are concretised in state action. In taking measures to deal with the poor the state expresses the common will, a set of expectations of how relations between individuals should be arranged and what the units of differentiation should be.

(Walton, 1983, p261)

Marx's response to Hegel is primarily (according to Colletti) at a philosophical level, criticising Hegel for collapsing everything into a predicate of the universal, that is, into the notion that the state is a manifestation of the realisation of the idea, rather than developing his ideas from empirical reality. As Marx notes, for Hegel, it is the state that creates all the movement in attempting to reconcile particular and individualistic interests. Marx in disagreeing writes that in reality the family and civil society are the precondition of the state: "they are the true agents....in speculative philosophy it is the reverse" (Marx, 1975, p62). What occurs in the Hegelian formulation then is an attempt to see the relationship between the state and civil society as in some sense contradictory, against this Marx is insistent that the state rises on the back of civil society and ensures its continuation by guaranteeing the existence of private property. As he writes: "The state stands in the same opposition to civil society and overcomes it in the same way religion overcomes the restrictions of the profane world i.e. has to acknowledge it again, restate it and allow itself to be dominated by it" (Marx, 1975, p221).

In asserting the general will and the equality of all, the state legitimises individualism and inequality.

Paradox reigns, therefore: the general will is invoked in order to confer absolute value on individual caprice: society is invoked to render asocial interests sacred and intangible: the cause of inequality among men is defended, so that the cause of inequality among them (private property) can be acknowledged as fundamental and absolute, Everything is upside down.

(Colletti, 1975, p37)

How then does this relate to the ideas and opinions of ancillary workers in the NHS. As indicated earlier, the notion that the state and through it the NHS, represents the whole community is one which can alter significantly the social intelligibility of political debate. Instead of questions about control and purpose becoming dominant, ones revolving around a sense of injustice become the point of articulation.

This is what lies behind Habermas' (1977) talk of a "legitimation crisis" where the role of the interventionist state erodes the spontaneous organisation of society and turns it into a world of deliberate decisions, which then takes fundamental political questions from the "natural" world of economics and into the more directly disputed world of politics. This makes the system as a whole more susceptible to crisis when a failure to deliver what has been promised occurs. However, whilst there may be a tendency within the process of reconstituting the state as representative of the organic whole to do this, what is of more importance is the role that this ideological formation has in intervening and redirecting ideas and opinions within society. It does this by allowing much greater stress to be placed on community-wide motivation as well as by making people think more directly about the effects of their actions on the community as a whole. It is ironic then, given Marx's strictures against the "citizen" that the advocates of counter-hegemonic struggle seem to be resurrecting this individual as the locus for their strategy.

Another complicating factor that stems from the operation of capitalism, and which intrudes between the trade union and the rank-and-file, is the acceptance of the commodification of labour by the workers themselves. This leads them to consider themselves as commodities with only their labour to sell and with other commodities to buy. A good example of this is the following statement from a male NUPE steward in Health Authority A:

In the end it's everyman's right to withdraw his labour and that's the ultimate, and it's everyman's right to sell his labour for what he feels he's worth, whether the market can stand it or not. If you feel that you're worth £20 an hour and the man gives you it - that is what you're worth. But the opposite way around is if the

122

government says you are worth ten pence an hour then its obviously their right to drive it down, as it is yours to drive it up, whether market forces can stand it or not.

(NUPE member, Health Authority A)

It is in this context that comments and beliefs about peoples' right to buy health care and to even cross picket lines (in the case of the NUPE member in Health Authority A) must be placed. The natural structure of competitive capitalism is a reified structure in which the relation between people becomes the relation between things. However, it would be wrong to believe that this tendency to reify only operates in one direction, because whilst it is true that reification is the natural response in civil society to the organisation of the state (in that everything takes on a "natural" appearance through the legitimation of the concepts of property etc by the state) and leads to individualisation; it is also true that such self- interested motivation is the reason for most of the actions taken by these health workers (and would be the reason, presumably, for any other groups taking action against competitive tendering). Thus, far from being a totally debilitating factor it has become an enabling one.

This does not mean that there is just a purely economistic consciousness at work, the actions of rational self-interest can easily flow (and do) into conclusions about class and politics in general. A good example of this was the strikers attitudes to the miners strike.

What this leads to, then, is a union committed to a non-market public health service, but with an active rank-and-file that partially accepts these ideas but limits them through the intervention of the concepts of organic community and individual rights. It would be wrong to leave things presented in this way though, because, in the same way that self-interest can act as an enabling factor, so too can these other concepts be capable of being refashioned into a partially counter-hegemonic form by the rank-and-file themselves. While it can be accepted that individuals have the right to buy health care and jump queues, it is also generally accepted that the market should have no role in the NHS and that things could be improved along welfarist "on the basis of need" lines. A G&M member at Hospital B talked approvingly of Germany as a model:

I was at a documentary the other day of Germany their national health. They call it the "twilight hours" of the elderly people, if they've got hip problems they jump the queue, if they've got to have their hip done so that their last few years is taken comparatively easily. Eye operations-they're immediately there for old people. Over here old people seem to be shoved to the back of the queue in England.

Within certain limits the effect of the ideological struggle waged by the union has had some positive results, even if these do not extend to questions of control or to alternative forms of social organisation. The way in which a notion of collectivism underlies their awareness of what could (or should) be brought about is in part subversive, given that we exist in a society which has never been able to meet all the needs present in it. Though this is very far from being an alternative world view, what it does show is the ability of the rank and file to remould and redefine concepts and ideas in terms of their own experiences and understandings.

Again, this is not without its negative aspect. As we have said ideology and opinion are not purely mental formations, they are also influenced by and dependent upon the activities that individuals are involved in. In a period when industrial struggles against privatisation seemed to go nowhere there were bound to be effects at the ideological level. These effects can vary, but with the emphasis that the union has put on the "moral" critique of privatisation, it has led to the ideological becoming more important than the industrial and hence cutting the roots of its own activity:

> I think at one time people were very union minded but over the past few years, some unions at the drop of a hat come out on strike and people have become browned off with it, like the motor car industry nd the miners, and the buses and the railways. If people are to catch a train somewhere and they're on strike it's not much of a joke because you could be losing money as well if you can't get to work. That type of thing, and I think people have got a bit fed up. At one time a strike was effective, it doesn't seem to be effective and yet people still strike and I think there's got to be some other example now, because strikes have had it. I don't think they've got the effect they used to have and all it seems to have done is put the members of the public against them.

Although this comment from a NUPE member in Health Authority A is probably atypical and extreme, it does indicate a certain trend towards the belief that industrial action (at least in the NHS) cannot win - and that other strategies have to be pursued. Even the militant NUPE official for Health Authority A had to admit that the focusing power of industrial action lay in the inconvenience that it caused the management, thus forcing him to prefer a cross-industry response to privatisation.

124

The importance of regarding industrial action in the way that this work has, is that it is based on the argument that without any form of activity, the educational and propaganda messages of unions like NUPE will fall on deaf ears; there being no focus on which to construct a counter-hegemonic ideology. Further, attempts to go beyond the confines of welfare statist, bourgeois democratic politics will also fail because people cannot just learn to take over institutions and control them, they have to do it themselves.

The conclusions that are produced by this piece of research are tentative but numerous. Firstly, the unions' approach to the the question of privatisation has to be assessed as ineffective. Here the unions' strategy can be judged in a very simple way; to what extent did it stop privatisation? Unfortunately, for the union as for the workers, the answer was a resounding No, the process of privatisation rolled on largely unaffected - turning its attention to other targets. However, at the level at which the strategy was conceived, it has had effect in influencing public opinion about the Conservative government's attitude to the NHS. So much so, that the issue of the NHS figured very highly in Labour's 1987 election strategy (as it did in 1992). As Michael Meacher, Labour spokesman on Health, said at the 1986 Labour Party conference: "the Welfare State and the NHS will be central to the next election" and so it was. But Labour still lost the election, why?

The answer to this connects with our second assessment. If the strategy was to be able to compensate for its rejection of economic means of opposing privatisation, then it had to have some assurance of success at an ideological level. The 1987 election proved that this was not so, for the simple reason that ideology is in essence contradictory and did not have one shape or form. Once all effort was put into winning over public opinion regardless of the circumstances in which it existed, it was very unlikely that the project could be successful. The main reason for this is that the position's misunderstanding of the ambiguous nature of public opinion[2] didn't allow for individuals to hold conflicting views.

In the same way that we have seen that contradiction is at the heart of the views of our sample of ancillary workers, so too, does it exist among the population at large. The view of Hall (1983) and of Golding and Middleton (1982) that there has been a tremendous rejection of socialism and of the welfare state among the mass of the population is overstated and simply not true. It posits the population at large with having ideological positions that are either one thing or another: laissez faire or welfarist.

As the work of Taylor-Gooby (1984, 1985a, 1985b) has shown there is considerable ambiguity among the public at large about the question of collective provision of welfare, with some parts being very popular (the NHS, old age pensions, etc.) and some not so (single parent and child benefits, council housing and low pay benefits). Similarly, alongside the widespread support for the NHS, there is also an acceptance of the role of and necessity for private medicine and private health insurance; concepts seemingly at odds with each other. These findings were confirmed by successive "British Social Attitude Surveys"(1984, 1985, 1986) during the mid 1980s. What this points to is, firstly, that reports of the death of support for the ideas of collective welfare provision were greatly exaggerated, and that secondly, this ambiguity coexists alongside major victories for the Conservative Party but do not account for them. Consequently, and to the great frustration of the Labour Party and its supporters, while the issue of the welfare state was accorded great priority by the mass of the population in opinion polls, and while it was also acknowledged that Labour has the best policies on these issues, it proved to be the case that this did not provide a sufficient reason for voting Labour. Thus it is that our group of ancillary workers have their connection with the Labour Party more because of its role in opposing the policy of privatisation than because of their acceptance of a coherent welfare state ideology.

The important point missing from the counter-hegemonic strategy is that it is impossible to recapture concepts such as "liberty" and "freedom" from the right, or even wage a moral campaign against them, if the material basis for such a hegemony is absent. The fact that people have what Gramsci described as "dual consciousness" suggests that individuals will have conflicting understandings of the world that they live in. This means that it is very difficult to wage a successful struggle purely at this level. The degree to which a person can tolerate incompatible ideas is considerable. Hence, the NHS ancillary worker who supports private health insurance. The basic failure of the counter-hegemonists is their inability to accept this ambiguity and the origins of it.

This ambiguity is not, however, static, its precise articulation depends on the power of the forces exerting influence on it. Within capitalist society among the most powerful of these forces are the ideas and ideologies of capitalism itself and the ideas and responses of the labour movement to them. Consequently, the terrain over which these contests were and are waged is the practical activity of ordinary people, that is, the activities that are pursued at work and in the home. Any attempt to change peoples' ideas in any genuine way is to a greater or lesser extent dependent on the state of social conflict. For it is within the practices generated by class antagonism that alternative practical forms of activities can begin to create a more coherent counter-hegemonic consciousness.

The question of building hegemony, therefore, is one of getting the ambiguous consciousness of the mass of people pointing in one direction rather than in the other, and for this the involvement in an aggressive and successful labour movement is essential; this is the only way of overcoming the inertia created by the atomisation that is the foundation of bourgeois hegemony.

The fact that the struggles against privatisation never became more than localised disputes in an era of trade union defeat provides reasons for the contradictory consciousness that the NHS workers displayed. Also, the fact that the trade union leadership took the course that it did and didn't stop privatisation shows the inadequacy of the strategy it was pursuing. Similarly, the failure of Labour in 1987 to win on the basis of highlighting issues like the NHS calls into question much of counter-hegemonic strategy.

We now move on to consider in more detail the arguments about the development of working class political consciousness in the post-war period.

Notes

1. This is not to support the Althusserian position of interpellation, where the individual is "hailed" as a subject by an all powerful social structure (Althusser, 1977). Giddens (1982) is right when he claims that this position is as functionalist in its implications as the work of Talcott Parsons.

2. Even the notion of such a thing as "public opinion" is highly misleading (see Roiser (1987) for a discussion). It implies a consensus of approach towards certain important political and social issues, and assumes that these are mutually exclusive to other approaches.

7 The Labour Party, the Labour vote, and the British working class

The purpose of this and the next three chapters is to broaden out the discussion of the theory and application of counter-hegemonic struggle to encompass wider theoretical questions such as the role of class and the nature of political consciousness. The previous chapters dealing with the ideas of the NHS ancillary workers were an attempt to show how in practice the counter- hegemonic positions did not work either reflect reality or succeed in their objectives. In this they were counterposed to a more radical form of combating privatisation and raising political consciousness; namely rank-and-file industrial militancy. This strategy by itself does not challenge the positions of what have previously been described as the "New Revisionism". These positions have stronger bases of support than just public sector trade union strategists. Furthermore, their influence extends further than just their own ranks and they have a capacity to influence the very nature of the "socialist project" itself, as well as how it could be achieved. Because of this, and with the evidence of the earlier empirical chapters, it is important to examine the areas where they feel strongest; namely, on the role, nature and influence of class in modern politics and on the nature of political consciousness. These two themes will be the basis for the final chapters of this work.

To start with class, one of the central arguments of the "New Revisionists" and one which underpinned much of their strategy was that of the irrelevancy of class and in particular the working class. These ideas manifested themselves in two separate but mutually reinforcing ways. Firstly, there was the debate about the effects of technological change on the composition of the working class in Britain from the second world war onwards. This focussed on its implications for working class culture, ideology, and activity, and in turn what this augered for socialist politics. Secondly, and intrinsically linked with this process in the minds of many commentators, was the seemingly downward spiral of electoral support for the Labour party. The structure of this chapter will be to look at three things; the composition of the working class; its electoral behavior; and the way in which these two questions can be the basis of an alternative conception of political consciousness.

Eric Hobsbawm, the working class and politics

This section will look at the work of Eric Hobsbawm, and in particular his essay "The Forward March of Labour Halted" (1981). This is an necessary starting point since in many ways it is here that the debate about the decline of class began, and to which reference is always made[1].

Hobsbawm began his analysis from the observation that by 1976 only 45% of the British working population could be classified as being manual workers. This figure had dropped from 75% in 1911, to 70% in 1931, and to 64% in 1961. The importance of this decline, for Hobsbawm, rested on the fact that during the nineteenth and the first half of the twentieth centuries the labour process was overwhelmingly dependent on manual labour, this had in turn led to the trade union movement being strong in areas where skilled manual labour was essential. It was these skilled workers who provided what Hobsbawm describes as the "backbone" of British trade unionism, and it was these same people, he argues, who were central to the development of the modern Labour Party precisely because of their trade unionism. It was not accidental that the Labour Party was preceded by the Labour Representation Committee (which was interested in getting any working person into parliament, irrespective of politics), or for that matter that the Labour Party developed out of the unions and not vice versa as happened with the SPD in Germany. The development of socialist ideology amongst trade unionists came at a later stage and was once again linked to their activity as workers and union members.

As the title of his essay suggests, the circumstances that brought about the creation of the Labour Party, and more importantly the Labour vote, were and are ones that depended on the fortunes of organised manual labour.

With the emergence of France, Germany, and the United States as rival economies to Britain during the early 20th century, the skilled worker found himself facing an erosion of his power. Far from being an irreplaceable part of the production process, what the new technology that had arrived with the increased competition threatened to do, was to turn him into an unskilled process worker, operating specialised machines or carrying out specialised parts of an increasingly elaborate division of labour.

Added to this was the development of a new tertiary sector of privileged clerical workers who saw their interests as being much the same as those of the middle class. This, Hobsbawm argues, produced a new form of labour aristocracy and eroded the superiority of the skilled worker. Another important factor in the widening of the gap between skilled worker and the middle strata was the role of the technicians and professionals who were drafted into the production process to manage the conditions under which everybody else worked. A process made worse by virtue that they were recruited from outside the boundaries of the shopfloor, rather than promoted from it.

In the face of such dilution, the skilled worker's response was to see his interests as lying with the rest of the working class claims Hobsbawm. As he goes on to write:

> The labour aristocrats were not only forced further away from the middle strata, but closer to the other strata of the working class, although their economic advantage (as distinct from their position in the social structure) was not seriously weakened before the First World War. They tended to be radicalised, especially in the great complex of industries in which mechanisation, mass production, and similar changes in the organisation of industry produced the most direct confrontation between the skilled worker and the new threats, in the growing complex of the metal working industries.
> (Hobsbawm, 1981, p7)

Though this did not mean that the working class had become a single homogeneous mass, it did mean that the working class had been drawn more closely together by a growing class consciousness, and that this had resulted in the creation of political demands in connection with education, health, and social security matters. Behind many of these developments was the emergence of what Hobsbawm calls the "common style" of proletarian life.

This common style, if I may so call it, of British proletarian life, began to emerge just about a century ago, was formed in the 1880s and 1890s and remained dominant until it began to be eroded in the 1950s . I am thinking not only of the rise of the socialist movement and the Labour Party as the mass party of British workers, the changes in trade unionism, the enormous and unbroken increase in the number of co-op members from half a million members in 1880 to 3 million in 1914, but of the non-political aspects of working class life - of the rise of football as a mass proletarian sport, of Blackpool as we still know it today, of the fish and chip shop - all products of the 1880s and 1890s : the famous cap immortalised by the Andy Capp cartoon, which is, broadly speaking Edwardian : and a little later, they had hardly developed much before the first world war, of the council flat or house, of the picture palace, of the palais de danse.

(Hobsbawm, 1981, p8)

It is within this context that Hobsbawm views the transformation of the British working class from one preponderantly manual to one in which the manufacturing sector is a minority. For him the working class as a cultural formation has disappeared. Alongside this change must be seen the shift that has occurred in the nature of capitalism, a transformation that is in part responsible for it. Hobsbawm is anxious to show that contemporary capitalism is marked by the dominance of state monopoly capitalism.

The factors which determine the workers condition are no longer, to any major extent, those of capitalist competition, The capitalist sector is no longer one dominated by the free market since it is largely monopolised, and the public sector both as an employer, and as provider of all manner of social services and payments, very largely determines them or at least the limits within which they are fixed. Political and not profit decisions determine it.

(Hobsbawm, 1981, p9)

This move away from competitive capitalism towards a state regulated variety (in an era of rising living standards and full employment) brought about qualitative changes in the unity and political awareness of the working class. While sectional differences within the working class such as those of locality or region, as well as those within the same industry, declined, what has increased are those divisions within the same level or grade. As Hobsbawm states: "It seems to me that we now see a growing division of workers into sections and groups each pursuing its own economic interest irrespective of the rest". This tendency he notes, is not limited to the traditional skilled versus unskilled demarcation dispute, but often has very little to do with technical qualifications.

This sectionalism is not confined in its effects just to where the conflict takes place, but also, due to the size and range of activities of the state, many such strikes directly affect other groups of workers, and argues Hobsbawm many strikes have this as an end:

> In fact it now often happens not only (as sometimes occurred even a hundred years ago) that groups of workers strike not minding the effect on the rest, skilled men on labourers, for example, but that the strength of a group lies not in the amount of loss they can cause to the employer, but in the inconvenience they can cause to the public, that is to other workers, by power blackouts or whatever. This is a natural consequence of the state monopoly capitalist system in which the basic target of pressure is not the bank account of private employers but directly or indirectly the political will of the government. In the nature of things such sectional forms of struggle not only create potential friction between groups of workers, but risk weakening the hold of the labour movement as a whole.
>
> (Hobsbawm, 1981, p14)

The thesis that Hobsbawm is putting forward is that with the transformation of the capitalist economy into its present form, the lack of any defined unity amongst the working class either by lifestyle or by work has led to sectionalism no longer acting as a cohesive force in the defence of working class living standards, but rather it has a fragmenting effect - in no small part due to the growth of the service sector.

On a more practical level Hobsbawm sees these changes as underlying a gradual erosion in absolute numbers of the Labour vote since 1951. This is because, he argues, support for the Labour Party is the political expression of class consciousness, and as the traditional manual working class has diminished, and as sectionalism has increased, the traditional bases for the Labour vote have declined. This tendency has become even more evident since the 1983 General Election where Labour received even fewer votes than in 1931. All in all it managed to get only 29% of the vote, 3% more than the newly formed SDP[2]. What was even more worrying for Labour was that amongst skilled workers Labour only managed to get 35% of their vote, and only 39% of trade unionists as a whole. Amongst first time voters 20% voted for the SDP as against 17% for Labour. Taken together the notion of a large working class vote for Labour seems to be a thing of the past. As Hobsbawm summed it up "The Labour vote remains largely working class, but the working class has ceased to be largely Labour".

It is in this context that we can see the connection between this line of argument and the New Revisionist orthodoxy. Hobsbawm, anticipating the likes of Mouffe and Laclau by a number of years, called for Labour to turn itself into the party of the people and to return to the halycon days of 1945. He suggests that then not only had Labour had the support of the working class, but was also "the party of all who want democracy, a better and fairer society, irrespective of the class pigeonhole into which pollsters and market researchers put them."

Class or class stereotype?

This interpretation, of British working class history and ideology does seem to come to the conclusion that class is not what it used to be. It suggests that the working class as a motive force in society is finished, capable at the most of indulging in the "economism" of industrial action over wages. In this way it provides an essential backdrop to the arguments of those advocating strategies of counter-hegemonic ideological struggle. For if the working class has become fragmented, sectional and economistic, then it is no good looking to it as the basis of socialist politics or even to stopping privatisation. This argument has been developed by some, notably Kitching (1983), to the point where the working class are the least likely to be interested in socialist politics given that they are the group most immersed in capitalist relations (i.e. pursuing economistic self-interest). Although, not all the positions subsequently developed out of his analysis can be attributed to Hobsbawm, the fact that he is the progenitor of this latest episode in the debate on the working class gives his views a special significance. A significance that demands an assessment.

One of the important aspects of Hobsbawm's work, as it affects this study, is his tendency to see class in purely cultural terms. This obviously echoes the tendency of other theorists to overstress the ideological dimension to class analysis (Poulantzas (1978), Hirst (1977)). Hobsbawm's analysis concentrates on the proletarian "style of life", its emergence, its decline, and its supercession. In these circumstances, it is useful to be aware that class, at least in more conventional Marxist analysis is usually seen as an objective relation to the ownership and control of the means of production[3] . This is not asserted as an article of faith, but rather to illuminate Hobsbawm's reinterpretation of class and the way it affects his analysis.

To turn now to the effect of the decline of manufacturing industry in

Britain on the composition of the working class, Miliband (1985), amongst others, argues that what has happened is not the decomposition of the working class but a recomposition. While this has been a complex process, in essence, all that has occurred is that the working class is now composed of different elements. Some of these are older, some are newer, but at the fundamental level of social determination it remains true that class exploitation and class potential still exist.

It is perfectly true that the working class has experienced in recent years an accelerated process of recomposition, with a decline of the traditional industrial sectors and a considerable further growth of the white collar, distribution, service and technical sectors. There is nothing particularly new about such a phenomenon: in one form or another, it has been proceeding throughout the history of capitalism, most notably, in the twentieth century, by way of of the truly dramatic disappearance of workers on the land as a very large component part of the working class. On the contrary, it is perfectly reasonable to argue that there has been an increase in the number of wage earners located in the subordinate levels of the productive process who, with their dependents, constitute the working class of the advanced capitalist countries and comprise the largest part by far of their populations.

This working class is not identical with that of a hundred or fifty or even twenty five years ago. But in terms of its location in the productive process , its very near limited or non-existent power and responsibility in that process, its near exclusive reliance on the sale of its labour power for its income, and the level of that income, it remains as much the "working class" as its predecessors. And so does that part of the population which is made up of unemployed workers, and of others, who are not in the productive process and depend wholly or mainly on welfare payments.
(Miliband, 1985, p9)

Similar points are made by Marshall et al.(1988) in their major study of the nature of class in modern Britain. Their arguments are all the more interesting given that their analysis is informed by a neo-Weberian perspective. They write:

...the current arguments suggesting that sectionalism, instrumentalism and privatism are somehow novel results of a recent restructuring of distributional conflict seem less than convincing. These arguments are the probable consequence of a tendency towards dualistic historical thinking whereby a communitarian and solidaristic proletariat of some bygone heyday of class antagonism is set against the atomised and consumer-orientated working class of today. Not only is it the case that historical data suggest a less romantic reality: sectionalism, privatism, and instrumentalism have always been close to the surface of working class life. It is also true that, conversely, class solidarities retain an importance that undermines many contemporary accounts of late capitalist societies in which sociability and altruism are reputed to have given way entirely to a "one-dimensional" and atomised consumerism.

(Marshall et al.,1988, p206)

While the empirical detail may always be the subject of debate, what is important are the processes of class formation and class antagonism. For it is these (the division of labour; the concentration of wealth and property in the hands of a minority; the competitive nature of the market; the priority of profit- making; etc.) that overdetermine the nature of any recomposition. If this is accepted, does this mean that Hobsbawm's argument falls? Not necessarily as at the centre of the Hobsbawm thesis lies a constant blurring of distinctions, and a consequent conflation of class with culture, and of both of these with political affiliation.

It is with this knowledge that the question should be reformulated by asking: "Has the forward march of labour halted?" Or perhaps would be: "What was the forward march of labour?" In the same way that Hobsbawm conflates culture and class and sees the working class as disappearing alongside the demise of the "Fish and Chip" shop, he also confuses the Labour Party and the labour movement. For Hobsbawm, the labour movement reached the peak of its forward march in 1951, a year unremarkable for anything apart from Labour receiving its highest ever vote. As Callinicos (1985a) points out, "The capital "L" is highly significant: the Hobsbawm thesis identifies the fate of the working class with the electoral fortunes of reformist parties" (Callinicos, 1985a, p131). Cronin (1984) also points out there is no necessary connection between class and political parties, as the early history of the trade union movement proves. The homogeneity that Hobsbawm assumes is not a natural one, but is in fact imposed on history in the interests of polemic. It is true that the working class, for much of the first half of the 20th century, attached itself politically to the Labour Party. However, these links were not automatic, as (is sometimes) implied by Hobsbawm, but had to be built up in the first place, and had (and have) to be constantly justified when Labour was (and was) in Government. The effect of this conceptual confusion is effectively to write off attempts to explain the history of the past few decades in terms of the understandings and activities of working class people themselves.

The evidence that these ideas are erroneous comes not just from theory, but also from the fact that they contradict the reality of the period. This can be seen from looking at the work of Cronin (1984), Panitch (1976), and Hinton (1984).

The homogeneity of the working class that is built into Hobsbawm's analysis is an aspect that separates him out from those others in the New Revisionism. For them, the whole idea that the working class could be a unified economic and political entity flows against the direction of their argument. It is probably for this reason that Wood (1986) omits all mention of Hobsbawm. However, as was pointed out earlier, the fact that Hobsbawm's own political development has its starting point in the Communist Party's popular front strategy of the 1930s means that he is very keen on strategies that call for the building of new hegemonic alliances. In this way he is at least a camp follower of the "New Revisionists".

The thrust of Hobsbawm's argument is constructed around giving a historical foundation to this position. Thus what occurs is the merging of the working class into the industrial working class, class activity into electoral activity, and class conflict into economistic sectionalism. Once this analysis has been accepted then the role for socialists is to construct alliances out of the divergent and semi-autonomous interest groups that are now the foundation of society. For Hobsbawm and the (then) Communist Party this is done through the "Broad Democratic Alliance". For others such as Hindess (1983) or Laclau and Mouffe (1984) it is done through articulating a radical discourse. In this way the importance of class is minimised (if not made redundant). Moreover, not only is class no longer central to politics, but more importantly those activities that are constituative of class are also accordingly downplayed, if not dismissed. Trade union activity becomes regarded as sectional and backward looking, existing mainly to perpetuate existing inequalities and extend them[4].

It is as an alternative to Hobsbawm's theory of the decline of the working class as a political force, that I wish to argue for a different analysis of the same history. This will be based not on the over-simple identification of class with party, but on the experience of the working class since the war. This means that I wish to leave the question of the falling labour vote until much later in this chapter, where it will be reintegrated into the overall argument. The explanation given will be one derived from the experience of members of the working class and not "from ambiguous facts helped along with a generous dollop of guesswork" (Westergaard, 1984, p78).

To start with it may be useful to quote from Stedman-Jones (1983):

> The whole idea of a forward march of labour is something of an optical illusion, or more specifically part of the social democratic mythology of Labour in the 1940s....If we are to understand the history of the Labour Party, we must understand it in terms of a number of discontinuous conjunctures which enabled it to achieve a particular and specific forms of success at widely separated points of time, rather than as a continuous evolutionary movement, which at a certain point mysteriously went into reverse.
>
> (Stedman-Jones, 1983, p243)

It is not only the history of the Labour Party that should be treated in this way, but also and more importantly the history of working class activity and consciousness because it is this which underlies it. During the period covered by Hobsbawm's analysis the structure of the British working class has changed and it has also gone through many different phases: from the wave of syndicalist activity that preceded, accompanied, and succeeded the First World War, to the defeat of the General Strike, from the economic prosperity of the 1950s and the 1960s to the stagnation and unemployment of the 1980s. Each of these moments brought about in differing ways differing political and ideological consequences. It is because of this that Hobsbawm's equation of economic militancy with the fragmentation of class consciousness is erroneous.

As Hallas (1980) points out, 1926 was a crucial turning point, both in terms of trade-unionism and for class consciousness for the labour movement. It represented the victory of a trade unionism which was primarily accommodative in character as opposed to one which saw its role as antagonistic to the economic rationale of capitalist society (a trend exemplified by episodes such as "Red Clydeside", "Red Friday", the election of A.J. Cook to the leadership of the Miners Federation of Great Britain etc.) If it represented an organisational defeat for the working class, then it also brought about an ideological transformation, allowing the possibility of a trade unionism that saw itself bound up in the corporate interests of the state[5]. The Mond-Turner talks of 1927 are an example of the explicit articulation of the ideology of class collaboration (Hyman, 1980, p65). Thus when looking at the period Hobsbawm concentrates on, from 1951 onwards it is important to be aware that its origins lie, not in the break-up of proletarian lifestyle, but in the changes in both practices and ideology that developed out of the defeat of 1926. Whilst it is true, as Hyman points out, that accommodation had long accompanied the activities of trade unions, it is also true that 1926 marked the sea change in attitudes that was to mark the post war years.

Developments after the beginning of the Second World War are marked by the emergence of what Jefferys (1979) describes as "national interest corporatism"; an ideological structure which formed the way the world was understood. Jefferys explains it in the following terms:

> Three ideas are crucial here, firstly, that the ideal form of corporatism is one where there is "voluntary" agreement between workers and employers on a common goal. Secondly, that nationalism, and especially war, was a crucial means of winning that "voluntary unanimity" between workers and employers such that the working class would "overcome" its "sectional" class interests. And thirdly, that "national interest corporatism"- the identification with the firm and/or nations interests is achieved at a price: workers interests must be seen to be "taken into account".
> (Jefferys, 1979, p2),

Why the war was so crucial in creating this corporatism was that for the first time the trade union leadership was seen to have a legitimate right to be involved in political decision making. At a more local level this process was even more marked, with the creation of Joint Production Committees within most sectors of productive industry. These committees, composed of representatives from both the workforce and management existed solely to optimise the output of what ever they were responsible for producing. In return for the co-operation of the workforce in these matters, the management was supposed to look good-naturedly at the complaints of its employees. By June 1944 over 4500 JPC's had been set up, covering 3 and a half million workers in factories throughout Britain. Whilst, as Jefferys argues, many of these committees were totally ineffective, they formalised the institution of shopfloor trade unionism as the dominant trend in the post-war labour movement. This move to the point of production was to have a dramatic effect in the years of prosperity that followed the war.

Before the war the local level of union organisation was dominated by the geographical branch or district committee. Workshop organisation was very patchy, and where it did exist, tended to be very weak. However, with the move to shopfloor organisation the power of the unions increased. The affluence created by the post-war boom allowed workers to take full advantage of their newly found power and produce the phenomenon of "wages drift". This is the habit of one group of workers after another attempting to force up their own standards of living by gaining an increase in wages over and above that negotiated nationally. This was usually accomplished by the tactic of the short "wildcat" strike in which a small section of a particular workforce would interfere with the running of the larger process until their demands were met. Consequently it was in this period, where continuity of production was paramount, that the role and influence of shop stewards grew - a factor that was to become increasingly important as the post-war boom turned into recession.

This argument describes the same development of sectionalism noted by Hobsbawm, complete with its attendant fragmentation of the working class, But instead of it having a negative character, it becomes, claims Jeffreys, constituative of the working class. The factors that Hobsbawm identifies as leading to the disappearance of the manual working class such as the growth of non-manual employment, and the state's changed role, are the ones that with the existence of shop-floor unionism led to a strengthening of the labour movement:

> It has been the survival and extension of this workplace based organisation that has enabled the manual working class to retain its' sense of common identity and to lock white collar workers into same reaction.
>
> (Jefferys, 1979, p10)

The effect of the post-war years was to "atomise" the working class: "Almost everything changed, the industries you worked in, the jobs you did, who worked alongside you, where you lived, how you lived, and what you thought about it all". What is suprising, comments Jefferys, is not the fragmentation, sectionalism, and separatism of the varied parts of the working class, but its continuity, resilience and relative homogeneity. It is this factor that he alludes to in his reply to Hobsbawm's "Forward March" thesis. He points out that white collar workers have become sufficiently proletarianised to be in the forefront of current unionisation. This has not been the passive unionisation of staff associations but has been based on the sectional interest militancy that has always existed in manual trade unions.[6]

As Stedman-Jones (1984) points out, the notion of self interested sectionalism at the expense of other sections of the community that Hobsbawm uses is one which is accurate when one is looking at the "winter of discontent" during 1978-1979 but develops major faults when applied to events such as the miners' strikes of the early 1970s, where instead of sectionalism, what developed was class solidarity among other sections of the labour movement not directly involved in the miners dispute (at least to some degree). Again, the political effects of the miners" strike of 1974 were the reverse of 1979. What is at fault in Hobsbawm's analysis is his belief that (at best) the working class is only capable of "economic" militancy, and that this is divorced completely from politics. Thus witness his remarks on the period 1970-1974:

...a movement is not necessarily less economist and narrow minded because it is militant, or even led by the left. The periods of maximum strike activity since 1960 - 1970-1972 and 1974 - have been the ones when the percentage of pure wage strikes have been much the highest - over 90% in 1971- 1972. And, as I have tried to suggest earlier, straight forward, economist trade union consciousness may at times actually set workers against each other rather than establish wider patterns of solidarity.

(Hobsbawm, 1981, p18)

Hobsbawm's notion of economism is one in which he sets a far too rigid separation between economics and politics. Engels wrote in "The Condition of the English Working Class" that strikes ·were the first attempt by workers to abolish the competition of the labour market, a competion that set them apart from one another. He also argued that strikes "imply the recognition of the fact that the supremacy of the bourgeoisie is based wholly upon the competition of the workers among themselves; ie, upon their want of cohesion. And precisely because the unions direct themselves against the vital nerve of the present order, however one-sidedly, in however a narrow way, are they so dangerous to this social order" (Engels quoted in Hyman, 1971, p6).

It was in this light that both Marx and Engels were to refer to strikes as essential in the creation of socialism, and it is for the same reason that later thinkers such as Rosa Luxemburg put such a high emphasis on industrial conflict.

Hobsbawm's dismissal of trade union activity as economism, in many ways exemplifies a criticism, made of him by Carlin and Birchall (1983), where in tracing the evolution of his thought they argue that nowhere in his work is there to be found the idea of working class self-activity. As a result, they claim, Hobsbawm's work often seems to lack a sense of struggle, past or present. Without this element, it is not surprising that his work abstracts in a hyperbolic fashion from impressionistic readings of sociological findings.

It is this concentration on the inter-relationship between economic and political activity that is central to Jefferys' thesis. Just as the post-war boom allowed the working class the privilege of indulging in "economism", so it was that with the gradual ending of the boom, the preconditions for this form of "do-it-yourself" reformism also started to disappear. The Wilson government of the 1960s appointed the Donovan commission in 1965 to look into what could be done to stop the "anarchy" of sectional wage bargaining. The conclusions it came to are instructive: it argued that wherever possible pay bargaining should be taken away from the shopfloor and be institutionalised at the level of the factory or company. This was to be accompanied by the greater use of more "formal" written agreements and procedures (designed in part to slow down the reactions of workers). Finally it wanted these negotiations to be widened to include new methods of work. Above all it wanted the whole enterprise to be predicated on the notion of "voluntary unanimity".

However in spite of these moves, the government and British capitalism in general was not capable of stopping workers taking action in defence of their interests. Not unconnectedly, it was at this time (late 1960s, early 1970s) that both Labour and Conservative governments attempted to add compulsion to their dealings with the trade unions. Both "In place of strife"(1969) and the Industrial Relations Act (1971) had as their objective the replacement of voluntary codes of conduct with legally binding ones. The result was the largest explosion of economic and political strikes that Britain had experienced for 50 years[7]. As Jefferys notes:

> For a time the chinese wall between economic and political industrial action was placed under siege. Fragmentation and sectionalism co-existed along side solidarity. Working class consciousness emerged among an active minority of workers with a political radicalism it had not possessed for two generations. Trade union consciousness spread rapidly amongst groups it had never touched before.
> (Jefferys, 1979, p23)

In many ways it is this concentration on the activity of workers that enables Jefferys to come to more optimistic conclusions about the possibilities of class-based socialist advance than Hobsbawm. However, the national interest corporatism talked about earlier does have some important negative effects on working class self-activity and these are probably (for the purposes of this research) of more significance. The most important one being the ability to harness the working classes' conception of its own interest to that of the capitalist class - this is done initially by the linking of workers pay claims to the profitability of the company in which they work. Therefore, whilst the years of the post war boom allowed workers to demand more and more from their employers, the effect of recession in the mid to late 1970s was to allow companies to argue that they have become uncompetitive, are making few profits, and need lower wages and less job demarcation. This in the majority of cases was accepted by employees and led to tremendous changes both in working practices and in shopfloor organisation.

Similarly the effect at the national level is illustrated by the effectiveness of the "social contract" constructed by Labour in the mid-1970s where the concept of the national interest was used to link the working class to the needs of the state - a link which ultimately damaged the economic interests of that class. It would be mistaken, though, to see these phenomena as purely the effects of ideology. The notion of the national interest much predates the Second World War and exists in countries that have very different working class traditions such as the USA. The fact that there exists in Britain a social democratic tradition that incorporates a nationalist element does mean that the working class finds itself limited by "economism", but not in the way usually argued.

In terms of understanding the processes of ideology this argument illustrates that individuals' ideas and understandings are not developed passively against monolithic structures (culture, institutions, etc.). On the contrary, they are based on real experiences in a changing world. This means that "economism" can become political and that the political (i.e. the Labour Party) can retard that development by constantly pushing people back into individualistic solutions.

The Labour vote - the parliamentary road to irrelevancy?

In turning to the question of the decline in the Labour vote from its high point in the 1950s, it is important to be aware of a criticism made of Hobsbawm's earlier work, and summed up forcefully by Westergaard:

> It sees the economic structure of class (or that part of it on which the argument focuses in order to claim that significant shifts have occurred) as in some sort of neat correspondence with socio-political consciousness. If the former changes, so in a matching way must the latter; and if the latter changes, there must be an underlying change in the former to explain it.
>
> (Westergaard, 1984, p78)

142

An argument that can be put forward as an alternative, is one that focuses on the relationship between the working class and Labour governments in power and which accounts for the de- partisanship of working class Labour voters in terms of this unhappy connection. However, before discussing this at any length it is valuable to be aware of the principle explanations of Labour's electoral predicament. These are interesting because the arguments they put forward bear striking resemblances to both the Hobsbawm thesis and the New Revisionism[8], in that they all argue that the working class has abandoned its socialism and that class politics make little sense (Franklin, 1986).

As if to illustrate this point McAllister and Mugham (1985) point out that during the 1980s, studies of British voting trends moved away from a concern with explaining the decline of the two party system to an emphasis on the ailing fortunes of the Labour Party. This was partly the result of the run of electoral defeats borne by Labour, but even in the early 1980s after only one such defeat this theme was present. The most eminent of these commentators, Ivor Crewe (1982), argued that Labour had suffered electorally because there had been a secular and long term erosion of support: "Labour now enters elections with a major handicap: unlike the Conservatives, its basic traditions run against the grain" (Crewe, 1982, p38). This he argued had become particularly noticeable since 1979, where principles that are traditionally associated with Labour served to further depress the Labour vote.

According to Crewe, in 1979 the main factor leading Labour supporters to fail to support Labour at the polls, was the effect of the "winter of discontent" of the previous year. Labour's association with the trade union movement was not an asset but a liability, at least in electoral terms. On top of this, on a whole number of traditional Labour policies, the electorate in general, and working class Labour partisans in particular had gradually moved to the "right" on each of them. Not only had traditional Labour voters become more like their Conservative counterparts in terms of specific issues, but they had also moved closer to where the Conservative party is perceived to stand on them.

The argument that traditional Labour voters had become estranged from the principles on which the party stands was also the starting point of Stuart Hall's influential "The Great Moving Right Show", where he argued that Labour lost the 1979 General Election because of the development of what he terms "Authoritarian Populism" which he describes as "an exceptional form of the capitalist state, which unlike classical fascism, has retained most (though not all) of the formal representative institutions in place, and which at the same time has been able to construct around itself an active popular consent" (Hall, 1983, p22). This ideological formation, which he and others saw as forming the basis of "Thatcherism", triumphed first in the Conservative Party with the replacement of Edward Heath as party leader (following the debacle of the 3-day week and the two miners" strikes of the early seventies), and then went on to win public support in the 1979 General Election.

The elements that constitute the theoretical side of this Authoritarian Populism (AP) originate in neo-liberal philosophy and free market economics. Both of these bodies of thought stress individualism and anti-statism and warn of the danger to society posed by Keynesianism and the idea of the welfare state. But as Hall points out "neither Keynesianism nor monetarism win votes as such in the electoral marketplace."

> But, in the discourse of social market values, Thatcherism discovered a powerful means of translating economic doctrine into the language of experience, moral imperative and common sense, thus providing a "philosophy" in the broader sense - an alternative ethic to that of the caring society.
>
> (Hall, 1983, p27)

Hall's argument fits in well with that put forward by Crewe and consequently provides the link with the New Revisionism, in that both seem to agree that there has been a fundamental re-alignment of ideology within the working class, or at least that section of it that used to vote Labour. Whilst Crewe charts this development (and explains it) in terms of attitudinal change, Hall is concerned to put it in the context of class relations within an advanced capitalist society. Hall's explanation starts from the belief that British capitalism has undergone a deep organic crisis which has forced it to go beyond being merely defensive in its efforts to defend the status quo. Instead, it had to go onto the offensive - "aiming at a new balance of forces". This necessarily involved the attempt to construct a new "historic bloc" of new political configurations and "philosophies". What occurred then, argues Hall, was not merely a political change in attitudes, but was in fact the creation of a radical populism. This succeeded in incorporating elements of peoples' own experience of the economic crisis of the 1970s into a "peoples' crusade", with its enemies being bureaucracy, union power, and statist socialism.

> When in a crisis the traditional alignments are disrupted, it is possible on the very ground of this break, to construct the people into a populist political subject; "with" not against the power bloc; in alliance with new political forces in a great national crusade to "make Britain

"Great" once more". The language of the "people" unified behind a reforming drive to turn the tide of "creeping socialism".
(Hall, 1983, p30)

Callinicos (1985a) has noted that in his later work Hall has developed this theme further so that it connects up with the work of Hobsbawm. Like Hobsbawm, Hall argues that the process of recomposition of the working class is one "likely to affect the industrial structure and political culture of the labour movement", therefore the decline in importance of the manual working class necessitates the labour movement to find other sources of support, because like other promoters of the New Revisionism, the working class, though analytically distinct from manual work, is still seen in terms of manual workers by Hall[9].

The convergence of so many of these arguments on the collapse of manual work in Britain has led the work of Hobsbawm, Hall, and Crewe to become accepted as an orthodoxy, at least on the left. However, although it is an analysis that seems to bear out the facts of industrial change and electoral decline, it is an argument that can be challenged.

Whilst it is certainly true that the culture and institutions that made up the working class style of life have gradually disappeared, and that these did give workers a common outlook and sense of identity; an identity which from the mid-1920s to the 1950s led them to vote in large numbers for the Labour Party. What is also true is that the break up of this common lifestyle did not automatically mean that they would cease to vote Labour. As Cronin (1984) in the course of writing about the debate over the "affluent worker" sees it:

What was missing from this argument, and from most of the attempts to come to grips with the 1950s and 1960s , was the recognition of the possibility of substantial material progress occurring within the existing class structure or, to put the matter more positively, of the fact that working people could take advantage of the new possibilities for consumption and make use of their new found prosperity without losing their sense of class awareness.
(Cronin, 1984, pp159-160)

What underlies many of these arguments is a form of functionalism which is concerned only with the effects of class structure and the impact of wage militancy and disregards the impact of Labour governments, themselves, on the people whom they were elected to represent. Cronin goes on to argue that the reason for the gradual break-up of the connection between class and party can be explained by the unravelling of the real links between the two after the Second World War and was further weakened by the fact that Labour failed to recognise the new situation and act on it[10]:

> Affluence would, of course have long-term effects. Over time, new forms of consumption and leisure would allow working people to by-pass some of the older institutions that had mediated between the class and the party, and help to loosen the links between them. But this happened gradually. This is not to deny the political impasse in which Labour found itself from 1951 to 1964, nor is it to minimise the evident failings of the unions over the same period. It is to suggest that the sources for these were to be located elsewhere than in the shifting structure of the working class or the supposed corrosive effects of social change. For the failures of Labour and the unions in these years had virtually nothing to do with the weakening of support from their traditional working-class constituents, but with their inability to advance to build up new bases of support and to attract new adherents... Nor was there any recognition of the potential for mobilising the increased material expectations and the growing sense of entitlement on the part of ordinary people behind a programme of structural reform. These were failures of omission, missed opportunities, and they were pre-eminently political failures.
>
> (Cronin, 1984, p172)

The forms of activity that the working class did involve itself in, on the other hand, were ones that were not only missed by the Labour party, but were actively combatted. In this sense Cronin is probably being optimistic in believing that Labour could have overcome its problems by trying to harness this energy. It would have had to choose between the working class and government. The link between the unions and Labour came close to breaking point during the late 1960s , when the Labour Government, having failed to deliver much over the previous few decades found itself in direct confrontation with the trade unions over incomes policy and produced the infamous "In Place of Strife" document. Cronin argues that this period "revealed the essential bankruptcy of the social democratic vision", because what was being presented by Labour was a rejection of the activities of the working class alongside a refusal to accept "the new sense of social worth" that was involved in the demands being articulated through industrial militancy.

The Labour Party, however, has had little to offer in the way of a political programme for the realisation of workers' enhanced sense of collective and personal worth. They have been lukewarm at best to the spread of shopfloor organisation and antipathetic towards what they see as troublesome wage claims. Towards the numerical strengthening of the unions they have been more favourably disposed, for obvious reasons, but towards the necessary acoutrements of union power - the independent power of shop stewards, the increase in industrial democracy, the politicization and democratization of corporate decisions - they have not been by and large sympathetic. In place of encouragement have come a flawed incomes policy, a restrictive industrial relations bill, and a savage deflation dictated by the International Monetary Fund and administered by the most recent Labour government.

In retrospect what is suprising about this contradiction between the trends of social change, opinion and action among working people, and the inert (or worse) response of the Labour party is not that it has led to a weakening of ties between Labour and the working class and, thus, between the direction of class formation and the evolution of politics. More suprising is the residual strength of the relationship, and the fact that so many working people still hope and work for a party that has so often failed to live up to the hopes and needs of its supporters.

(Cronin, 1984, p14)

The existence of what has been characterised by Callinicos (1985a), amongst others, as "the changing locus of reform"[11] has ensured that in the long term the activities of the working class run directly into contradiction with the political/electoral success of the Labour Party. The working class could continue to raise its standard of living only to the extent that British industry had control over the markets it was competing in, and could still make a profit. As long as this happened they were prepared to tolerate this situation of increasing wage costs. The 1960s, however, saw the beginning of the rise to ascendancy of Japan and Germany in world trade. With such competition, British industry was forced to take up the question of labour productivity, and as a consequence had to try hard to stop "wage drift" and break rigid demarcation in working practices. The Labour party was therefore caught between two stools, wanting to stay in Government, and wanting to represent the working class. One pressure demanded the need to respond clearly to the lagging behind of British industrial production by increasing the productivity of labour, while the other pushed them to defend workers from the consequences of this drive for higher productivity.

147

Panitch (1976) describes this situation as being one where Labour's simultaneous role as both an integrative and representative institution in society came into conflict. And it is this feature of the Labour Party that has had more to do with Labour's electoral decline than any other. The problem as Panitch sees it is that, "Labour's frame of reference is not primarily focused within the orbit of the working classes" subordinate position in British society.... These considerations are not absent from Labour's conception of its role, but they are confined within a national frame of reference - a concern for national unity shared in common with Britain's dominant classes - in which the aim of making Britain's economy viable is paramount"[12](Panitch, 1976, p235). As a consequence, though Labour's power (especially in electoral terms) is derived from the working class, it uses this authority, not to make demands on the employing classes, but to further integrate the working class into the social system. In effect, it plays the role of an agent of social control, constantly mediating between class and nation.

What Panitch has outlined, though accurate, is not very different from any number of critiques of social democracy advanced from the time of Lenin onwards. However, what is interesting about Panitch's argument is the way in which he accounts for the processes which lead to this development, namely through the use of the concept of corporatism. Though by no means an original notion[13] (witness the earlier discussion), corporatism, when used by Panitch, can account for some of the behavioral characteristics exhibited by Labour governments, when in power. This can be added to the argument advanced by Jefferys earlier, in which the power of shop floor led reformism was also limited by its reliance on a form of corporatism. It is in the combination of these arguments that we can more fully account for the weakening of Labour's hold over the voting habits of the working class. For whilst Labour can only be effective as an integrator to the extent that it "represents" the working class, the working class responds by accepting much corporatist ideology and identifies its interests with those of the nation.

As stated earlier, this is not to say that it is only the existence of the Labour party that ensures the maintenance of national interest corporatism in the working class. It obviously comes from many sources, but the fact that much of the working class (both then and now) looks to the Labour party as its political representative means that this world outlook has immense power. Insofar as this is also the point of view and attitude of the the trade unions, the same is true of them too. However, in order not to paint a too one-sided picture of the situation, it is also the case that whatever the nature and power of the ideology, it cannot of, and by itself, contain all situations. This is illustrated by the example of the now infamous "Winter of Discontent", which not only involved health workers, but which centred on the assertion by many groups of workers of the right to free collective bargaining after almost a decade of differing sorts of incomes policies. While the Conservative attempts at wage restraint had foundered on the rocks of legal compulsion and trade union power, Labour had been far more successful by getting voluntary agreement from the unions for their social contract and ensuring that the unions themselves policed any outbreaks of militancy. The end result was that even the power of the call for national unity was not strong enough to stop a rank and file rebellion in the face of record rates of inflation. Accordingly the policy fell and so did the government.

So far the connection between the working class and the Labour vote has been described in very broad terms; talking either of an ideological abandonment of social democracy by large sections of the electorate, or of a continual failure of the Labour party to represent the class that it expects allegiance from. Whilst the weight of evidence tends to correspond to the latter, this of and by itself does not make the former any the less convincing. What is needed is some reference to empirical studies, though it hardly needs stating that there are few facts in the social sciences and that all evidence must be treated critically.

As was pointed out earlier, in this field it is almost regarded as a truism that Labour was suffering from an ideological catastrophe, as more and more working class people abandon the values of socialism. McAllister and Mugham (1985) argue that the evidence of the 1979 General Election does not support the conclusions made by Crewe and others. From a statistical re-analysis of both the 1974 and 1979 British Election studies they conclude that there was no disproportionate decline in the attitudinal belief of Labour supporters along the 4 themes that they identify as comprising Labour party doctrine; "these are socialism (nationalization and government control of building land); class interest (the redistribution of wealth and introduction of comprehensive education) internationalism (the reduction of defence expenditure); and trade union power" (McAllister and Mugham, 1985, p45).

Thus they argue, that whilst there was an indisputable decline in the strength of attitudinal socialism among both Labour partisans and the working class, this decline was more or less of equal magnitude among Conservative partisans and the middle class. The reason for Labour's defeat at the polls was "a generalised reaction against the policies, performance, and promises of a party that had to steer Britain through difficult times, both at home and abroad". The 1979 election was notable for the effect on voting made by issues that cut across and overode socialist commitment "and thereby encouraged the defection of certain working class individuals who would have probably otherwise remained loyal to the Labour Party at the polls". These issues were principally race relations and law and order. As the authors point out, the fact that these issues were relatively new on the political scene, as well as that they can hardly be argued to constitute traditional Labour principles, meant that Labour could only be affected at the polls. What they do not point to is evidence of Labour's inexorable decline. Two observations are made by McAllister and Mugham:

> The first is that, to the extent that issues did independently influence the voting decision, they did not do so uniformly for the two parties. In the case of the Conservative party, all the issues in fact served to reinforce fidelity among both the parties identifiers and the middle class. In other words, the independent effect of issues was always to cement party loyalty by complementing supporters attitudinal structures rather than contradicting them. The Labour party by contrast, enjoyed mixed fortunes in that some issues prompted loyalty and others cut across the socialism of the parties support groups, especially the working class, and there by encouraged defection. It is clear, therefore, that issues in general can only have redounded to the Labour party's disadvantage and the Conservative party's advantage in 1979.
>
> (McAllister and Mugham, 1985, p49)

To this evidence can be added the work of Heath, Jowell, and Curtice (1985) which also concludes that there has not been a substantial fall in the working classes" indentification with Labour. This again may seem contrary to the evidence, but as they point out, most work on voting behaviour borrows directly from the classification of class developed by market researchers, and is more interested in spending power than in economic relationships. Consequently, there is a failure to distinguish clearly the work situations of respondents. The self employed are distributed among all the classes in spite of them having a distinct class position and interests of their own. Similarly, working women lose their own separate identity and become subsumed under the classification of their husbands.

By redefining the categories of the market researchers into ones which distinguish more adequately between routine work and the opportunity for control over it, the authors conclude that there is no evidence of significant class dealignment since the 1960s. The perceived weakness of Labour amongst the skilled working class has arisen because of the lumping together of foremen, technicians, and the manual self employed, with skilled workers, who have little or no control over their daily working lives. When separated out, this group shares many of the same political attitudes as unskilled workers.

Thus in a "normal" election (as opposed to the one in 1983, where Labour lost among all classes) Labour should be able to bring out its traditional class vote, even though those who could be described as working class on this redefinition only comprise 34% of the 1983 electorate in contrast to the 47% that they represented in 1964. This still means that Labour has been weakened by the gradual decline of this traditional working class insofar that low grade white collar workers do not automatically look to Labour as their party.

The answer to the question of why Labour have done so disastrously in the last two elections lies, for Heath, Jowell and Curtice, in the combination of the social and political levels of determination:

> On the one hand social class housing, education and other aspects of social structure constitute the sources of group interests. These interests provide a basis for political action. On the other hand, the political parties may help to shape group values and foster an awareness of their interests. They can influence the extent to which the potentials are realized. It is the interaction between the social and the political that determines how people vote.
> (Heath, Jowell and Curtice, 1985, p10)

The conclusion that they come to with this analysis is the unremarkable one that the Labour voter was dissatisfied with the policy of his or her party in the 1979 and 1983 elections. Thus the Labour vote slumped. The strength of this position does not lie in its statement of the obvious, rather its power stems from its non-acceptance of the structural determinist account of voting behavior. As argued above, while class still has explanatory power in understanding voting patterns, politics is also of prime importance. If a party is not seen to be representing its supporters" interests fully then its support will decline. Consequently, they argue, the only way to arrest the Labour Party's electoral decline is for it to articulate the interests of the working class more fully. This, they suggest, can be done by stressing social equality as the principle around which the Labour party should operate.

The salience of social class in voting behavior is also strongly underlined by Marshall et al. (1988). Agreeing with the work of Heath and his colleagues they call into question some of the methodological techniques used by the supporters of class de-alignment most noticeably their class categories. Like Heath et al. they prefer to use a class schema based on the work of Goldthorpe. Using it they also identify the importance of politics in explaining Labour's unpopularity at the polls:

> Our data suggest that Labour voters in particular respond to the language of social class and see the world around them structured by class processes. It would seem, then, that Labour gains to the extent that it succeeds in constituting and mobilizing class interests by presenting issues in class terms, and reinforcing the formation of collectivities with common class identities. The fact is, of course, that the Labour Party and trades unions alike have been relatively unsuccessful at mobilising members in precisely these terms, especially when compared wth their counterparts in countries such as Sweden, Austria and Norway.
>
> (Marshall et al., 1988, p254)

As they write "cynicism and disillusionment" among working class Labour supporters are more important in explaining Labour's voting record than any structural reason.

That there was nothing pre-determined about the effect of social changes on the Labour vote was illustrated by figures published in "New Society" (September 26th, 1986) which suggested that under the leadership of Neil Kinnock, Labour had regained most of the working class support that it had lost in 1979. This trend was especially noticeable among the skilled manual vote whose loss in 1979 was the foundation of much of the debate about the disappearing Labour vote.

The importance of economic prosperity in underpinning electoral support has been put forward as a crucially determining factor by a number of writers. Sanders and his colleagues (1987) downplay the "Falklands Factor" that is popularly seen as providing the Conservatives with their 1983 election victory, and instead emphasise the importance of perceived economic prosperity. They see the variables that affect the elector-as-consumer (personal taxation, consumer spending, interest rates, and short time working) as having a direct influence on personal expectations and that these expectations constitute "the single most important direct influence on government popularity" (Sanders et al., 1987, p313). Following up this analysis Sanders (1991) claims that "movements in government popularity during the 1987-90 period can be predicted remarkably well from a knowledge of just two independent variables: the level of personal economic expectations (lagged by 3-4 months) and the interest rate (lagged by one month)" (Sanders, 1991, p241). The implication of this argument are that the outcomes of electoral contests are very dependent upon circumstantial factors which only affect small numbers of the electorate. Consequently the role of third parties is critical. The success of the (then) Alliance parties in the 1987 General Election took considerable pressure off the Conservatives, while their disarray in the late 1980s gave Labour considerable succour and put them in a position to challenge for government.

It is important that Labour's third election defeat is seen in this light, if for no other reason than to show that Labour need not be consigned to electoral insignificance - at least for this reason. Goran Therborn (1984) provides more evidence to justify this optimism by placing Labour's (then two) defeats in their international context. In a survey of the prospects for socialist advance in advanced capitalist countries, he listed 8 countries in which the labour movement had topped 50% of the vote in national parliamentary elections since 1965. In Austria, France, Greece, Portugal and Spain, this had occurred since 1976, and 1981 was marked by this happening in both France and Greece, countries where victory for the Left had either never happened before, or had been a generation in coming. This is all the more impressive when it is considered that in all these countries the size of the industrial working class was either diminishing or did not have the social weight that it has in Britain.

Again what this seems to indicate, is that there is nothing pre- ordained about the connection between social structure and political allegiance, and that what matters are the conjunctural aspects of the political scene in a particular nation state.

What we can conclude from this discussion of Labour's electoral record and the international comparisons is that working class voters were acting more pragmatically in the face of the reality of social democracy and the renewed economic prosperity of the 1980s. The complicating factor in Britain for Labour is not that it has lost its working class support for ever, but that the Conservatives can provide certain sections of the working class with short-term tangible benefits, whilst for others the emergence of the Alliance as a credible force has stopped the natural movement back to Labour among all classes. Working class voters (and especially white collar ones) now have to be convinced of the benefits of a Labour government in competition with the policies of the Conservatives and Liberal Democrats. The absence of any successful labour movement struggles (the miners' strike, the print workers" and ambulance workers" disputes, etc.) has also meant that the working class has not been provided with any foundation on which to reject individualistic pragmatism.

That the Labour Party at a national level has sought to distance itself from these events has further compounded its weakness given that it is only through the strength of the labour movement that it has any influence. This is particularly important given that, as Stedman-Jones (1984) points out, Labour electoral victories have always depended on a large influx of non-working class votes in order to win. To reach these groups demands that the working class as a movement is going forward. To use Gramsci's terminology non-fundamental classes have to be articulated to one or other of the fundamental classes. They are incapable of political leadership on their own.

Because of this political failure, in the circumstances of the 1979, 1983, and 1987 elections the attraction of Labour to many white collar workers simply was not present, this when added to the substantial number of manual workers who simply did not vote Labour made the Labour vote apparently crumble. In the circumstances of an assertive labour movement it is likely that significant numbers would follow its lead. The victories of 1945 and 1974 would seem to indicate this.

The question of Authoritarian Populism

If the psephological argument is open to interpretation then this must also make us question the validity of Stuart Hall's analysis of Thatcherism, and especially his assertion of the working classes' ideological incorporation. Apart from what has been noted above, Bob Jessop and others have posed some important questions concerning the coherence and accuracy of the Authoritarian Populism (AP) thesis. They argue that one of its major faults is its capacity to mean different things to different people. As they say; it "appeals to the left because it condenses a large number of interpretive schemes and can be stretched in different ways according to circumstances". Depending on circumstances, either the authoritarianism or the populism is the element stressed. The other main fault that they point to, and the more important one, is its "ideologism"; that is its excessive concentration on the ideas that keep the Conservative's in power to the exclusion of any discussion of the contradictions and tensions that exist within Thatcherism. Consequently, like many of the electoral studies looked at earlier, what is assumed is that "the "message" as emitted is identical to the message as "received and understood"".

The AP approach correctly notes that the Tories provided appealing explanations for the failure of Keynesianism, offered a means to express resistance to the defects of bureaucratic welfarism, legitimated the individualising experience of work in modern capitalism, etc. But

154

it does not establish which of these messages, if any, were accepted and by whom. Thus the AP approach tends to homogenise the impact and universalise the appeal of Thatcherism.

(Jessop et al, 1984, p38)

As they go on to ask, "are anti-statist themes as resonant in the conservative assault on the Health Service as in the attack on nationalised industries?" The answer is obviously not. Underlying the homogenisation of the AP approach is a belief in the "exaggerated unity of the Keynesian Welfare State and its social democratic character". In other words the AP approach tends to see the welfare state and Labour as inextricably connected. It ignores not only the fact that the welfare state owed more in design to liberalism than to the Labour party, but also the significance of "Butskellism" and "MacWilsonism" in the 1950s and 1960s . Thus what Jessop et al. are arguing is that Thatcherism, whilst certainly representing a break with the terms of the post-war settlement, did not necessarily mean an utter transformation of ideology. Firstly many of the elements making up the ideas of AP have been long present in popular ideology - both Conservatives and Labour have at different times used elements in their approaches to both domestic and foreign policy. If there was any novelty in Thatcher's ideas, they argue, it was in the fact that they more closely corresponded to grassroot Tory opinion than had been achieved before.

Even in the articulation of her ideas Mrs Thatcher was not prepared to take them to their logical conclusions. For example, she did not argue for a full bodied neo-Liberal approach to the welfare state - instead she advocated a 'social" market economy and moved cautiously in tackling key elements of the welfare state. Hence the privatisation of domestic services but not of medical care. While much of this is related to a fear of going too far, part of this caution can be related to the fact that the Conservative Party depends on two groups for its electoral success - the deferential voter and the pragmatic secular self seeker. The conclusion Jessop et al. draw from this distinction is that Conservative support is a function of on the domination of AP ideas in the population as a whole, but rather rests on a combination of traditional voting (which do include elements of AP ideologies but which also pre-date the emergence of Thatcherism). This is joined with the pragmatic self-interest voting of various individuals searching for lower direct taxation, lower inflation, council house sales, etc.

This, in light of the Conservative Party's failure to organise the working class politically (the lack of influence of Conservative trade unionists etc.) as well as the volatility of the working class vote, means that the basis for

Thatcherism and hence for AP was not that strong. As they write "there is no single ideological or organisational basis of Thatcherism and that its success depends on other factors, including luck" (Jessop et al, 1984, p43). They could also mention the opportunism of the Conservatives in promoting council house sales and give-away de-nationalisation share offers.

If, as the evidence seems to suggest, neither the long term decline of the manual working class, nor the ideological incorporation of the electorate is an adequate explanation for Labour's electoral decline, and if the importance of economic class is not rejected, then a satisfactory explanation must accept that voting Labour is not the only form of class consciousness possible. Because social democratic governments, once in office, are forced to act against the class they purport to represent, then constant support for them cannot always be achieved. Conversely, it must also be concluded that the link between workers and Labour has not been broken for all time, but that for the moment people see a disparity between ideals and practice. Consequently, people will vote according to what they perceive as being in their best interests in much the same way as they have always done and for some this will mean acting as privatised consumers. To quote Therborn (who was writing in the left-wing nadir of the early 1980s) on the prospects for socialist advance in Britain:

> The prevailing sense of gloom certainly has a basis in reality, but the main point is that the political and ideological crisis or bewilderment of the socialist left has to be located in a broader historical framework of overall labour movement growth, increased assertiveness, and actual advance. Otherwise our moorings in historical reality will be broken by a tide of momentary impressions and experiences.
> (Therborn, 1984, p18)

Discussion of the impact of "New Revisionism" on accounts of class and electoral politics in Britain during the 1980s has been wide ranging. This has been necessary because in their various ways, the debate over class, the argument over the nature of post-war industrial militancy, and the question of Labour's seeming electoral decline all interconnect and feed into one another and provide the base for the hegemonic politics outlined earlier. In questioning these assumptions on their own ground it is possible to challenge the whole of this new orthodoxy's position.

If it is the case, as I have argued, that the working class cannot be subsumed under the category of manual labour and that in turn the industrial activity of workers is not just a "bloodyminded" economism pursued by otherwise "selfish" individuals for the worst of motives; then these ideas are operating on different ground to those whose work has been criticised. Moreover, this theory of how ideology operates in society changes from one based on various forms of discourse theory to one based upon reflexive subjects.

Similarly, the fact that members of the working class seem to hold apparently contradictory ideas and are often to be found supporting right-wing ideas is not an immense theoretical problem heralding the collapse of socialism as an ideal, or as something dealing the death blow to cherished forms of political activity. Rather, these factors can be understood as stemming from the essential nature of capitalism; its competitiveness and its production of alienation, and from the fact that no institution in society exists to counteract and challenge capitalism effectively. It would be naive to expect class consciousness and political direction to develop purely out of numerical strength. In this way analysis comes to focus on the question of political organisation. Discussing the need for a party of one sort or another in the process of turning the working class to socialism and advancing social change, Panitch makes the following observations:

The whole point of inserting the working class party into the equation as a mediating factor between class and socialism - and putting it less abstractly and formally than equations allow, the historic importance of the forming of "mass" working class parties around the turn of the century - was precisely that they were more than the electoral aggregators of individual expressions of pre-existing class identity, projecting them into the state arena as conduits for the attainment of governmental office by party leaders (socialist or otherwise). Mass working class parties were rather the essential condition in the twentieth century for the reinforcement, recomposition and extension of class identity and community itself in the face of a capitalism which continually deconstructed and reconstructed industry, occupation and locale. They were the essential mechanism for the transcendence of sectionalism, particularism and economism not only through the national identity given to the class through its association with the party's project of winning state office, but through their potential role in socialist education and mobilisation. After all, if the notion of a hegemonic class project means anything, if the struggle for socialism was to be more than elitist, vanguardist, a war of manoeuvre (pick your anti-Leninist adjective), then it above all required class identity and community of a new kind. This had to include widespread understanding of how capitalism worked in general, of why supporting a workers party meant being against capitalism as a system, and of a socialist vision that meant more than "more" in the particular and economistic sense, all leading to a self-confidence on the part of a very great number of working class activists to provide leadership in their wider communities in relation to multifarious forms of subordination, deprivation and struggle.

That the Labour Party has not played this role has a great deal to do with the impasse of working class politics.
(Panitch, 1985, p64)

Class consciousness, therefore, becomes the most important ingredient in the political mobilisation of the mass of the population. This differs considerably from the perspective of the "New Revisionists" in that, for them, it is the articulation of a discourse that is most important. Implicitly this rejects the notion of human activity as being of any major importance - given that in their schema language and ideology are primary. Class consciousness on the other hand, involves the articulation of existing economic conflicts onto a political plane.

This can only be done by a political organisation involving itself in the day-to-day activities of the working class. As Marshall et al. point out: "Between the perception of common interests or consciousness of shared values, and joint pursuit of these in co-ordinated action, lies the necessity of collective action" (Marshall et al., 1988, p259). This does not necessarily mean that it comes in and imposes its ideas on the working class, but rather that it takes the healthy and politically progressive ideas and practices of the class and develops them in a systematic and anti-capitalist way. It is this that is closest to Antonio Gramsci's notion of hegemony. For it is widely forgotten that Gramsci regarded his work as attempting to ground the Leninist concept of political organisation in Western European surroundings. His idea of building hegemony was one of winning the working class to anti-capitalist socialism not just creating a "democratic discourse" for the existing state.

To conclude then, the effect of the New Revisionism on political practice has been extensive. However it is one that is based on a form of crude economic determinism which demonstrates itself in the form of its understanding of class. It is also one that ignores the reality of peoples' lived experiences in relation to class conflicts and electoral politics. The result of this is that it not only fails to account historically for its conclusions, but even more importantly, is incapable of providing an adequate political strategy for the tasks that confront it.

Notes

1. Even though he does not share many of the theoretical conclusions of the New True Socialists, his being an older political trajectory influenced by 1930s Popular Frontism, it is still correct to list him among the protagonists of the new orthodoxy given his close connection with the journal "Marxism Today".

2. These figures are all from Hobsbawm (1981).

3. See for example the famous passage in "The Holy Family" which makes it explicit that it is class position that matters, not what individuals do or think (in Marx and Engels, 1975, p37).

4. For an interesting account of this perspective in the field of welfare provision see Weatherly (1988).

5. For a fuller discussion of the importance of corporatism on British society see Middlemas (1979) and Panitch (1976).

6. This is a contentious issue provoking much debate, see Carter (1985) for an overview. Wright (1985, chapter 5) also has some interesting things to say on the nature of class and on political consciousness.

7. For a fuller account of this period see Crouch (1979).

8. Indeed, Miliband (1985) refers to the "Crewe-Hobsbawm School of Psephology" (Miliband, 1985, p65).

9. So much so, that in his talk to the "Gramsci 87" conference organised by Marxism Today he talks of the end of the "proletarian moment" (Marxism Today, June 1987). Hall also provided many of the underpinnings for the ideas of "New Times" such as "post-fordism" etc.

10. Similarly, Panitch (1985, pp57-67) is also led to conclude that what underlies the current "impasse" of social democratic politics is not so much the decline of the traditions of the manual working class but the failure of the Labour Party to continually renew its links with the people that it purported to represent.

11. The term refers to the ability of workers to directly change their own standard of living without recourse to parliament or "politics". In this way, "reformism" as a strategy is circumvented.

12. Panitch has dealt with the question of Labour's dual role at greater length in his "Ideology and Integration: The Case of the British Labour Party", (1971).

13. The sense in which Panitch uses it is also different from its more general usage (see Schmitter, 1974), rather it is concerned with the incorporation of the working class into the capitalist system and not with the processes of decision making that occur with the breakdown of political pluralism. These are also the issues that interest the collection of essays bought together by Jacobi (1986). Also see the essay by Cameron in Goldthorpe (1984).

8 Ideology 1: Structuralism, post-structuralism, and Marxism

The concern of this chapter will be to develop theoretically the conclusions outlined in previous chapters. We have seen how the ideas held by the interviewed group of ancillary workers are contradictory in relation to the welfare state. We have also seen that there has been a gradual erosion of working class electoral support for the Labour Party and that this trend has been linked to the behavior of Labour when in office. The argument I have been trying to develop, therefore, is that a contradictory consciousness is the nature of most peoples' understanding of the world. This explains why the group under study had seemingly incompatible ideas about the provision of health care. This "dual consciousness", however, is not fixed for all time, rather, it is unstable and prone to change. It is for this reason that the nature of the post-war working class and its relation to politics was discussed. For, it is through the practical activities of a class that the precise balance of dual consciousness is constructed. The failure of the Labour Party to adequately reflect that activity and facilitate it, has meant that the balance has shifted in the direction of individualism and consumerism. Thus it is entirely compatible for NHS ancillary workers to be against privatisation and for private health insurance.

This brings us on to the second part of the research, namely, the relevance of counter-hegemonic strategies in the response to privatisation. As has been pointed out before, the theory of ideology

161

(whether explicit or implicit) that provides the inspiration for this view is one which accords primacy to ideas and as such is invariably influenced by structuralism. We have seen its' inadequacy at a practical level in its failure to successfully win over those most affected by privatisation, now I intend to look at its intellectual roots and show how a properly constituted theory of dual consciousness is superior to it at a theoretical level as well. Such a theory will argue that the epistemological relativism and decentred nature of structuralism leads to a misrecognition of the processes of ideology and thence to faulty political conclusions.

Structuralism and its impact on theories of ideology

Structuralism as a theory can be said to originate with Ferdinand de Saussure and his posthumously published work "Course in General Linguistics". Here, in opposition to the orthodoxy of the day, Saussure argued that language was more than just a naming process. By this he meant that there was not a simple object - word correspondence. Rather, a word was related to a concept rather than to an object. The importance of making this move was that it introduced into linguistics the notion that the concept (the signifier) was completely arbitrary in relation to that which it represented (that is, there was no necessary resemblance or correspondence between a sound-image and the thing represented). Furthermore, he also argued that the process of signification depended more on the relations holding between the units making up the language than on the reality that it represented. These relations are ones based upon the concept of "value". To explain what he meant by this Saussure gives the example of money: to understand what a particular coin or note is worth, we must be aware of how much of a particular commodity it can be exchanged for, and that it is also possible to compare it with a similar amount of money in the same currency.

> In the same way a word can be exchanged for something dissimilar, an idea; besides, it can be compared with something of the same nature, another word. Its value is therefore not fixed so long as someone simply states that it can be "exchanged" for a given concept, i.e. that it has this or that signification: one must also compare it with similar values, with other words that stand in opposition to it. Its content is really fixed by the concurrence of everything that exists outside of it. Being part of a system, it is endowed not only with a signification but also and especially a value, and this is something quite different.

Saussure's linguistics has at its core the notion that the differential relations between concepts is the foundation of language. As he writes: "Whether we take the signified or the signifier, language has neither ideas or sounds that existed before the linguistic system, but only conceptual and phonic differences that have issue from the system. The idea or phonic substance that a sign contains is less important than the other signs that surround it" (Saussure, 1966, p118).

The importance of this development is brought out by Callinicos:

> Language, therefore, for Saussure, consists in two parallel and interdependent series, the signifiers and the signified. Each series is constituted by the relations between its elements, sounds and concepts respectively. These relations and the elements themselves are produced by difference. One can see here the starting point for some of Saussure's most well known themes - notably his insistence on the priority of "langue","the whole set of linguistic habits which allow an individual to understand and be understood", over "parole", its usage in speech, and of synchrony, the relations constituting "langue" at any one time, over diachrony, the evolution of language. It is in this sense that Saussure is called the father of "structuralism" - he regards the system of difference constituting "langue"as the privileged level of linguistic analysis.
>
> (Callinicos, 1982, p29)

This account of the formation of language has made its effect felt far outside of the field of linguistics. The reason for this, argues Callinicos (1982), is that it has challenged the ascendancy of the "subject" in philosophical debate. The traditional theory of language held that the meaning of a word resided in an entity outside of language and to which the word referred. The security of this relationship is provided by the subject who orders the world through his or her consciousness. Under the structuralist linguistics of Saussure, language no longer resides in an extra- discursive reality, it becomes autonomous of it. Similarly, the subject is now no longer the source of meaning and in this way becomes the result of "certain relationships which both were prior to and exceeded it" (p30).

Benton (1984) also acknowledges this shift when he writes that instead of the subject being the bestower of meaning, it has become its "prisoner". Once achieved in linguistics, this radical decentring of the subject, has been adopted in a variety of other disciplines. This has happened most notably in France where the functionalism of Compte and Durkheim has always provided a pole of opposition to the subject orientated philosophies of existentialists such as Merleau-Ponty and Sartre.

One of the most significant thinkers to take up and extend the ideas of structuralism was Claude Levi-Strauss. His essentially anthropological studies attempted to use the model of structural linguistics to account for such social phenomenon as kinship and myth. This was not done without some modification of Saussure's original ideas. As Anderson (1983) points out, Saussure himself had specifically warned against the extension of his theories to explain kinship and economics. "Saussure's whole effort, ignored by his borrowers, was to emphasise the singularity of language, every thing that separated it from other social practices and forms" (pp 42-43). Against this warning Levi-Strauss' structuralist anthropology saw kinship systems as a kind of language and all social activity as a form of communication. The departure from Saussure's ideas that this argument entailed was the one of giving primacy to the signifier over the signified. As has been pointed out earlier, in Saussure's linguistic model, language is seen as consisting of two parallel series, the signifiers and the signified (sound images and concepts). These are completely integrated with each other and cannot be separated.

Levi-Strauss' model breaks this connection by arguing that because there is a superabundance of signifiers in relation to the signified, the result is a surplus of signification, and accordingly a dislocation between the two series of signifiers and signified. What is meant here, is that because language contains an infinity of sounds that were all created together (language, to be a language must arrive complete, or it does not have the status of language) then, there are going to be sounds with no real referent. These, Levi-Strauss describes as "floating signifiers" and it is these that give rise to new meanings. The relations governing the signifiers (and thus the production of new meanings) have priority over the signified. As a result, Levi-Strauss is able to argue that the symbols are more real than that which they symbolise.

Similarly, the French psychoanalyst Jacques Lacan, has also promoted the idea that the signifer is more important than the signified. Working in the field of Freudian theory, Lacan has challenged the notion that the unconscious is the product of repressed biological instincts. Instead he argues that language is fundamental to the development of the human individual. As Eagleton (1983) writes:

In gaining access to language, the small child unconsciously learns that a sign only has meaning by dint of its difference from other signs, and learns that a sign presupposes the absence of the object that it signifies. Our language "stands in" for objects: all language is in a way "metaphorical", in that it substitutes itself for some direct, wordless possession of the object itself. It saves us from the inconvenience of Swift's Laputans, who carry on their back a sack full of all the objects that they might need in conversation, and simply hold these objects up to each other as a way of talking. But just as a child is unconsciously learning these lessons in the sphere of language, it is also learning them in the world of sexuality. The presence of the father, symbolised by the phallus, teaches the child that it must take up a place in the family which is defined by sexual difference, by exclusion (it cannot be its parent's lover) and by absence (it must relinquish its earlier bonds to the mother's body). Its identity as a subject, it comes to perceive, is constituted by relations of difference and similarity to the other subjects around it. In accepting all of this, the child moves from the imaginary register into what Lacan calls the "symbolic order": the pre-given structure of social and sexual roles and relations which make up the family and society. In Freud's own terms, it has successfully negotiated the painful passage through the Oedipus complex.

(Eagleton, 1983, pp166-67)

Leaving aside the question of whether or not this is a valid re-interpretation of Freud's ideas, what is important in Lacan's account is the role of language in the creation of absence and exclusion. Following traditional Freudian theory Lacan sees the effect of the Oedipus compex as leading to a "split" subject forever divided between the conscious ego and repressed desire. However, the 'real" exclusion from the mother leads the subject to involve itself in the endless process of difference and absence that constitutes language. As Eagleton explains: "the child will now simply move from one signifier to another, along a linguistic chain that is potentially infinite" (Eagleton, 1983, p167). It is this continual movement from signifier to signifier that creates desire which is in essence a lack which humans strive to fill. Language thereby severs humans from the "real" and replaces it with an incompleteness that cannot be overcome. There can be no "transcendental signifier".

The result of Lacan's psychoanalytic structuralism was to further weaken the connection between the signifier and signified. This occurred because, in Lacan's scheme, it is not the case that both of these parallel series are each determined by differential relations between their elements. Rather, what occurs is that the signifier becomes the series that makes up langue while the signified becomes the series that makes up parole. What this means is that the signifieds can only be the outcome of the play of the signifiers - "...the concrete uses to which the differential relations constitutive of language (= langue = the signifier) are put" (Callinicos, 1982, p38).

When combined with his emphasis on the fluidity of language (substitution, metaphor, metonymy etc.) the effect is, Callinicos argues, to make language into an endless play of meaning with no external referent to establish its validity. Consequently, the effect of Lacan's work is to radically break the connection between reality and language or at the least slide the signifier under the signified.

This tendency becomes more explicit in the work of Jacques Derrida who adapted Saussure's concern with the distinction between langue and parole and between synchrony and diachrony into a position where there can be no series of independently existing signifieds. He argues that Saussure's notion of the inseparability of the signified and the signifier is at odds with his acceptance of the signified as a determinant idea or meaning. Thus, argues Derrida, Saussure allows for the existence of a concept independent of the signifier. For Derrida on the other hand, there can be no "transcendental signifieds". Meaning can only be created in the play of difference in the play of signification[1]. Thus writing becomes more important than the spoken act. This is because writing, as marks on a page is dependent on its spacing for its intelligibility. It is thus more systematic than the spoken word which is affected by temporality and context. Derrida's position is summed up by Giddens (1979) in the following terms:

> Derrida's work can thus be seen as giving a new impetus to Saussure's formalism at the same time as it disavows the connection of that formalism with langue and synchrony: substance or the "concrete", is repudiated both on the plane of the sign (rejection of the transcendental signified) and on that of the referent (an objectively given world that can be "captured" by the concept). For each of these, which may be said to approximate respectively to idealism and positivism, Derrida substitutes the productivity of chains of signification.
>
> (Giddens, 1979, pp30-31)

The effect of structuralism on Marxism.

The influence of structuralist thought on Marxist theory has been profound. Often described as the "revolution of language" (Callinicos, 1982, p48), the conclusions put forward by the structuralists and post-structuralists, if accepted by Marxists create serious doubts about the adequacy of Historical Materialism as a social theory and as a scientific project. The work of Derrida is an instance; for him, all knowledge, including that of the social world, can only be a discursive knowledge constructed within language. Given language's lack of an external referent, any knowledge produced can only ever be a knowledge of language and never of the realities of which it wishes to speak. This not only causes fundamental problems for Marxist epistemology (where a real world is accepted as existing), but also provides the basis for a non-materialist examination of power and ideology in society. Hence, out of post-structuralist linguistics we get the emergence of the work of Deleuze and of Foucault with their emphasis on knowledge as power.

The work of this pair, especially of the later Foucault, has been important in grounding post-structuralist ideas in the discourses of empirical reality. This is significant given that Foucault's earlier work had been dedicated to the "archaelogy" of systems of thought (epistemes) such as medicine in which truth is relational to the period and tasks with which it is involved (Foucault, 1973). Insofar as they did so their focus remained at the cognitive level (Harland, 1987), however Foucault's later work on penal systems and sexuality takes a shift to materialism; to power over bodies and to controlling their actions and activities. Foucault's insistence on the importance of establishing the "geneologies"(which relate to power and are transgressive) rather than "archaologies" of particular knowledges establishes them as social practices and according to Dant they "become enmeshed in a politics of discourse" (Dant, 1991, p130).

In his later work Foucault established that power is not just a political phenomenon but is in fact a crucial aspect of everyday life. In this scheme of things power is not merely focused in certain institutions but is pervasive throughout the whole of society producing a multiplicity of points of resistance. As Hewitt points out:

Rather than concieve of [power] as extending downwards from some central point, headquarters,ruling caste, economic elite, or soverignty, Foucault sees it immanently as originating from below in each instance of the machinery of production, in families, groups, and institutions. It is this conception that informs Foucault's account of the development of bio-power, its embodiment (in "force relations", "the body" and "the social body") and its instruments of application (the disciplines and technologies of regulation, the "panopticon", the "carceral"and the "tutelary complex"). Each of these figures is examined in turn. Whilst power is studied in ascending order from its local to its global formations, whether state, law or ideology, the analytical focus at each level remains the force relation. This relation is neither one of unchanging domination nor of total submission of one party to another. It is dialogic, exhibiting the never equal and yet ever mobile play of dialogue.

(Hewitt, 1983, p70)

Central to the whole model is knowledge, because it is through knowledge that the use of power can be negotiated. In other words, reality and power can only be understood in the context of the articulating practices surrounding discourse. Politics is thus the conflict between different discourses.

Structuralism and its discontents

The influence of structuralism over Marxism stems in the main from the lack of a theory of language in Marxism itself. Therefore structuralist analysis has filled this absence with its own ideas and has brought its own epistemological baggage with it. While this is not the place to discuss all the various Marxist solutions to this problem, we can point to some absences in structuralist theory. Firstly, as Giddens points out, the arbitrariness of the signifier is not something that stands up to close examination. Giddens argues that Saussure conflates the signifier with the real object itself but only talks about the arbitrary nature of the sign in the context of the signifier / signified relationship. Consequently, there is no discussion of the world of which the signifier speaks. "Ideas or concepts participate in the process of semiosis by combining with signifiers; but how ideas or concepts achieve any capability of referring to objects or events in the world is completely unexplicated" (Giddens, 1979, p15-16). The crux of Giddens's argument is that Saussure has no theory of the competent speaker or language user. Once this is acknowledged, the heart of structuralism and post structuralism is removed in that the competent subject interferes with the free play of the signifier by attempting to root it in contexts and understand them.

Anderson (1983) in a similar light points to three principle difficulties underlying both structuralism and post-structuralism. The first he describes as the "exorbitation of language". Drawing exclusively on linguistics structuralism and its antecedents accepts as given a "totalizing and dialectical reality anterior and exterior to the consciousness and will of any speaking subject, whose utterances on the contrary are never conscious totalizations of linguistic laws" (Anderson, 1983, p44). That this asymmetry is erroneous is indicated for Anderson for three reasons. Language changes slowly and unconsciously; utterances have no material constraints, are not subject to scarcity, and in normal circumstances have little effect on social structures; and finally they are axiomatically individual. All in all, borrowing from linguistics removes collective agency from all the spheres in which it is applied.

The second difficulty he points to is the "attenuation of truth" this he sees as proceeding from a "gradual megalomania of the signifier" as structuralists have repressed the referential axis of Saussure's theory of the sign to the point where Foucault can claim that truth is a tyranny we can well do without. This removes any need for evidence to be verified in any discourse and undermines any objective of rational knowledge.

Anderson's third objection to structuralism lies in its "randomisation of history". Because there is an unbridgeable gulf between the general rules of syntax and the use of any particular sentences, history from a structuralist perspective has to be understood from position of "langue" that is its conditions of poossibilty. The result is a massive effort directed at classification rather than explanation. Causality is a casualty of such procedures and historical explanation based on contingency as structural movement becomes the product of chance.

To quote Anderson: "Diachronic development, in other words, is reduced to the chance outcome of a synchronic combinatory"(Anderson, 1983, p50). In the light of these points it would seem that structuralist accounts are inimical

Marxism and language

The Russian formalists and in particular V. N. Volosinov started rolling the ball of providing a foundation for a Marxist understanding of language in the early part of the 20th century. Volosinov, working in post-revolutionary Russia published his "Marxism and the Philosophy of Language" in 1929. Within it he argued that the Saussurian model of linguistics rested on a separation between the system of rules that constituted langue and any practices located outside that system. This was improper on two counts he felt; firstly it did nothing to explain how language was used in practice; and secondly, as a consequence, it could only deal with variation within a language and not its' determination. Thus the structuralist model could not explain linguistic use or change other than that which occurs through the structure itself. As has been pointed out above, the human subject is again missing, a disturbing omission given that the whole purpose of language is communication.

Again, the solution is the reintegration of the synchronic and the diachronic, that is reasserting the primacy of human action in the use of language.

> The sign, in its actual and concrete usage, is thus always socially formed. Its actual use and meaning, in the case of language, is reciprocally determined by whose word it is and for whom it is meant. It is always set within and, in part, moulded by a particular set of social relationships between speaker and listener: that is, by particular conditions of socio-verbal interaction which are themselves moulded by the broader social, economic and political relationships in which they are set.
>
> (Bennett, 1979, p79)

In this way linguistics can be rooted in the practice of human subjects, rather than in the autonomy of the structure of language itself.

Callinicos (1985b) in assessing the problem of language and historical materialism moves in a similar direction to Giddens and Volosinov by attempting to root language in a truth conditional theory. Such theory owes more to Anglo-American analytical philosophy than to Marxism, but, according to Callinicos it provides a realist account of language that is not narrowly representational by basing itself on the way that we use words to talk about the world. In other words the need for a sentence to satisfactorily explain the world is an important part of language. As a result sentences must fit together with the rest of a language in a formal (logical) pattern in order to facilitate this process. Consequently, language is both a formal structure and a basis for a realist epistemology.

Structuralism and Marxism

That there is an incompatibility between Marxism and Structuralism can be seen by the post-war developments in French intellectual life. After an initial period of fraternisation between the two schools (the structuralist Marxism of Althusser, Balibar, Ranciere, etc.) the tensions started to create splits that eventually led many Marxist intellectuals into embracing the political Right. Among those who have taken such a path are such respected figures as Andre Glucksmann, a student and co-thinker of Louis Althusser, who has become in many respects the leader of the "nouveaux philosophes" who orientate themselves explicitly against Marxism. Their main distinction has been the reformulation of the Marxism = totalitarianism thesis so beloved of the Cold War ideologues.

This, in and of itself is not particularly suprising, every generation of radicals produces its" own renegades. What is suprising is the adoption of these ideas by Structuralist but otherwise left-leaning thinkers. When reviewing a book of Glucksmann's, Foucault also concurred with his conclusions. He wrote:

Stalinism was the truth, "rather" naked, admittedly, of an entire political discourse which was that of Marx and of other thinkers before him. With the Gulag, one sees not the consequences of an unfortunate error but the effect of the most "true" theories in the order of politics. Those who hoped to save themselves by opposing Marx's real beard to Stalin's false nose are wasting their time".
(Foucault, quoted in Callinicos, 1982, p108)

In other words Marxism is not only just another discourse, but it is in fact a dangerous one, possibly more dangerous than the discourses of capitalism. Marxism is incompatible with structuralism as much politically as theoretically. As in the similar case of Freudianism, attempts to incorporate Marxist theory with structuralism, necessitates one or other of the theories coming out on top. There can be no real synthesis fair to both sides, only unstable amalgams. This is proved by looking at the history of such syntheses[2]. All of them have proved theoretically unstable (a look at the number of auto-critiques and self- criticisms proves that) and most have ended up justifying the kind of political conclusions that traditional Marxism is completely opposed to. Laclau and Mouffe's radical democratic discourse is just a more recent twist.

Subsequently, the epistemological relativism and decentred nature of structuralism is one that needs to be rejected if Marxism is to survive as a theory. And it is the purpose of this study to argue that it is in the adoption of structuralist derived arguments that we get a misrecognition of the processes of ideology and thus faulty political conclusions.

However, the awareness of this problem is not very high amongst most Marxist writers on ideology. Most Marxist accounts of ideology attempt to bring in at some level a degree of structuralist reasoning. Unsuprisingly, this is most noticible in work influenced by the Althusserian tradition which has favoured the dominance of structure over the activities of acting subjects. This has in turn affected the way in which ideological processes are viewed.

A major conflict within Marxist theories of ideology is that between active conceptions and passive conceptions. Favouring the former I will be arguing against the rejection of the subject implied in structuralist accounts and for one which recognises the acting subject.

Notes

1. *"Differance* is thus a structure and a movement which can only be grasped in relation to the opposition of presence / absence. Differance is the systematic play of differences, of traces, of the spacing whereby elements are connected with one another" (Derrida, quoted in Giddens, 1979, p31).

2. It is in this light that we must see the various attempts to create a structuralist Marxism (Althusser and Balibar, Hindess and Hirst,Laclau and Mouffe, etc.). Each of them in their turn has tried to use the principles of structural linguistics as the basis for Marxist analysis (Althusser with his notion of "structures in dominance", Hindess and Hirst and their typology of modes of production,Laclau and Mouffe and their "radical democratic discourse"). The attempt to engage effectively with structuralism on the part of Marxists has generally been deemed a confusion and a failure (Thompson, 1978; Anderson, 1983; Callinicos, 1982, 1985b).

9 Ideology 2: Social practice and the role of the subject

As with most concepts heavily used in Marxist theory, the term ideology has no single definition. The treatment it receives in the works of Marx and Engels is perfunctory rather than complete, and as a result of this, all we are offered is a fragmentary collection of ideas on the subject rather than a completely articulated concept. This has made use of the term problematical and has led to a myriad of interpretations all attempting to be "true" to the founding texts. As McCarney (1980) notes:

> The task of explicating Marx's view of ideology is one which, notoriously, gets no systematic attention in his own writings. Indeed, for all the use made of the concept there is little that may safely be taken even by way of oblique comment on its grammar. We are given a set of clues and left to discover the pattern for ourselves.
>
> (McCarney, 1980, p1)

Partly as a result of this, and partly due to the nature of Marxism as a politics, the discovery of this pattern has become a major growth industry within Marxism during the last century, All the important figures of 20th century Marxism - Lukacs, Gramsci, Althusser, have each attempted to develop out of Marx and Engels' work a systematic concept of ideology. However, because each has also insisted on taking a distinctively different approach to the question there has been no overall agreement on the conceptual status of the term, with the consequence that there are as many theories of ideology as there are Marxist approaches.

Before posing a Marxist theory of ideology in opposition to that of the discourse theorists, an awareness of this profusion of Marxist theories of ideology is necessary. At the same time it is important not to be overwhelmed by it. Rather than attempting to explore the whole body of Marxist work on ideology, emphasis will be given to themes that are relevant to this study such as the role of social structure in Marxist analysis and the linked question of subjective consciousness.

To understand fully how these two themes interrelate in discussions on ideology it is first necessary to trace out Marx's philosophical development. Studying at the Universities of Bonn and Berlin during the 1830s Marx was fully immersed in the traditions of Hegelian idealism which, during that period, had reached the status of an official orthodoxy. Central to the ideas that Marx took from Hegel at this time, and which he was to use throughout his later studies, was the notion of dialectical change. For Hegel, History was the history of change and these changes occurred because of the contradictory nature of thought and reality[1].

While it was true, that for Hegel, this whole process was concerned with the unfolding to philosophy of the absolute idea, what was also true about his method was that the process also stressed the importance of human agency in transforming the world.

It was this "practical" dimension to Hegel's work that particularly attracted Marx, and he, along with the other "Young Hegelians", saw Hegel's philosophy of change as a justification for the democratisation and liberalisation of German society. In asserting this reading of Hegel, Marx and his co-thinkers were responding to the conservatism of Hegel's more orthodox followers who saw the creation of the Prussian state as the culminating point of history - in that it was the embodiment of the "Absolute Idea" and represented the highest form of freedom. It was this political split in Hegelian philosophy as well as the limitations of the Young Hegelians" position that sparked off the development of Marx's materialism and his eventual rejection of Hegel. This process was by no means automatic and depended crucially on the intervention into the debate made by another Young Hegelian - Ludwig Feuerbach.

For Feuerbach the major problem with the Hegelian system was its inversion of the processes of the dialectic. It stressed the centrality of ideas in determining historical change. To correct this Feuerbach proposed to give the dialectic a foundation in reality. In the Hegelian system, the moving principle of the dialectic was man's estrangement from the absolute idea (God) which was embodied in Nature. What developed out of this process was a religious teleology in which History was a movement towards the point where man could overcome his alienation from Nature by virtue of his realisation of the dialectical process itself. In other words, History was a process whereby the existence of the Absolute Idea could be acknowledged and Man's reintegration into Nature confirmed. In realising this, Man - or at least the Hegelian philosophers - would become the identical subject-object of History. Both being a result of the development of History and at the same time being aware of how historical change occurred.

Feuerbach, on the other hand, argued that the dialectical nature of History was the result of man's estrangement from Nature and not from the absolute idea:

> This speculative feat was, according to Feuerbach, a reflection of an inversion at work in reality itself. Man's estrangement from himself: the evolution of human consciousness led to the creation by the imagination of an alien being to whom all man's essential powers were attributed.
> (Callinicos, 1985b, p29)

This led Feuerbach to stress that the foundation of the dialectical nature of reality was human beings themselves and not God. Moreover, he argued, what Hegelian philosophy had done was to invert the natural order of things. But if this was a materialist rendering of the dialectic, it was still one bound up in the teleology of estrangement, alienation and ultimate reconciliation, and was therefore idealist in form if not in content. Marx, adopted these ideas and used them initially to buttress his radical Hegelianism. This gradually gave way to a fully fledged materialism in which the imperative of social change was not the overcoming of alienation (from God or nature), but the overcoming of the contradictions inherent in production and thus in society. This process was slow to develop and was not completed for many years[2], but slowly Marx started to conceive of the class nature of production as being the cause of all social contradictions and the source of Man's alienation from society. The work of Feuerbach had been central to this intellectual development insofar as it redirected Marx's efforts into looking at production and thus enabled him to discover the working class as an agent of social change.

The method by which Marx came to these conclusions was as important as the conclusions themselves. Larrain (1979) writes that Marx's early thought sought to combine two elements. 1) a philosophy of consciousness and, 2) a scientific rationality in regard to the material determination of reality.

> From the philosophy of consciousness Marx draws the idea of the active subject, but this subject becomes historically concrete. The Kantian consciousness as such and the Hegelian "folk spirit" are replaced by the historical class and its practice. From the new scientific rationality Marx takes the concern for material reality as the real starting point of science and the critique of religion, but this material reality is conceived as historically made by men and, therefore, susceptible to be changed by their practice.
> (Larrain, 1979, p35)

Thus Marx writes in his first thesis on Feuerbach:

> The chief defect of all hitherto existing materialism - that of Feuerbach included - is that the thing, reality, sensuousness, is conceived only in the form of the object of contemplation, but not as human sensuous activity, practice, not subjectively. Hence it happened that the active side, in contradistinction to materialism, was developed by idealism - but only abstractly since, of course, idealism does not know real, sensuous activity as such. Feuerbach wants sensuous objects, really differentiated from the thought object, but he does not conceive human activity itself as objective activity. Hence, in the Essence of Christianity, he regards the theoretical attitude as the only genuinely human attitude, while practice is conceived and fixed only in its dirty-Judaical form of appearance.
> (Marx quoted in Engels, 1978, p65)

Here, the conclusion that Marx took from his studies of Hegel and of Feuerbach was that consciousness of the world is inextricably linked with practice in that world. By practice, Marx is referring to the continual creation and re-creation of social life by human activity. Central to this reproduction of life is the process of production and the ensuing social division of labour. This is by definition a collective and co-operative activity leading in turn to the development of institutions and social relationships which are not freely entered into. Consequently, these structures constitute an "objective power" over which men and women seem to have little control. Paradoxically, practice can also be liberating; in that by their own actions men and women can alter these social relationships through, what Marx describes as, "revolutionary practice".

It is in this context that the concept of ideology is formed. For, if the notion of practice plays a crucial role in the formation of ideas then consciousness should reflect that practice. However, if the practice is a practice of an incomplete reality then ideology will be produced. Accordingly, ideology is to do with those ideas which do not describe or account for reality correctly. This is to say that there is an epistemological dimension to the concept of ideology.

If this is the ontological side to the early concept of ideology developed by Marx in "The German Ideology" then its other side, in which Marx talks about the ruling ideas in any society being the ideas of the ruling class, is the side which illustrates more fully its critical nature. Here, the division of labour which brings about the creation of classes gives to the dominant class control not only of the means of material production but, also, access to the means of mental production. This results in both an intellectual hegemony for the dominant class (in terms of what ideas are generally accepted) and a dominated classes inarticulacy (in that it finds it difficult to articulate its own interests because the ideas it uses express the interests of its oppressors). The importance of this aspect of Marx's conception of ideology lies not in its establishment of a genetic link between ideas and a class, but in the acceptance of the fact that ideological ideas express the interests of a dominant class. Marx delineated the two elements of a theory of ideology that he went on to use throughout his intellectual career and which distinguished the ideological from the general determination of ideas. Larrain (1983) sums this up:

> For Marx, therefore, ideology does not arise as a gratuitous invention of consciousness which purposefully misrepresents reality, nor is it the result of a conspiracy of the ruling class to deceive the dominated classes. The distortion which ideology entails is not the exclusive patrimony of any class in particular, though ideology serves only the interests of the ruling class. That all classes can produce ideology is the consequence of the universality of the "limited mode of activity". That ideology can only serve the interests of the dominant class is the objective result of the fact that the negation or concealment of contradictions plays a major role in the reproduction of those contradictions: it is only through the reproduction of contradictions that the ruling class can reproduce itself as the ruling class. To this extent, the reproduction of contradictions can only serve the interests of the ruling class. So the role of ideology is not defined by its class origin but by the objective concealment

of contradictions. This is achieved by trying to reconstitute in consciousness a world of unity and cohesion.

(Larrain, 1983, pp28-29)

If what we have outlined above is how Marx conceived of the notion of ideology then we must be also aware of its partiality and instability.

> The problem Marx faces in building a new theory of consciousness is twofold: how to reconcile materialism with the fact that reality should not be conceived as a given object which does not include the subjects activity; and how to reconcile idealism with the fact that being cannot be reduced to thought. While materialism makes consciousness a reflection of external reality, idealism makes reality the product of consciousness. Materialism splits into two separate worlds what Marx thinks to be a unity whereas idealism dissolves one world into the other.
>
> (Larrain, 1979, p38)

As Larrain (1979) in an earlier work pointed out, there is a conflict between the idea of the individual as subject and the idea of the individual as object which is never really resolved. Consequently, instead of one unitary theory of ideology developing within Marxism, we have instead two general notions:

a) ideology as distortion
b) ideology as reflection

a) emphasises the role of consciousness in creating ideology whereas b) is more concerned with the effect of structure on consciousness. If the derived ideas of commodity fetishism and false consciousness are examined it can be seen how these different concepts can fall into one or other of the above positions.

The concept of commodity fetishism was one developed by Marx in "Capital" to account for the fact that capitalist material practices are not capable of being understood purely by subjects just experiencing them. The real character of practice is concealed by distorting appearances that are constitutive of reality itself. This problem of phenomenal forms is particularly acute in the economic sphere of the circulation between commodities. In a famous quote from "Capital" Marx wrote:

> The sphere of circulation or commodity exchange, within whose boundaries the sale and purchase of labour power goes on, is in

178

fact a very Eden of the innate rights of man, it is the exclusive realm of Freedom, Equality, Property and Bentham. Freedom, because both buyer and seller of a commodity, let us say of labour power, are determined only by their free will. They contract as free persons who are equal before the law. Their contract is the final result in which their joint will finds a common legal expression. Equality, because each enters into relation with each other, as with a simple owner of commodities, and they exchange equivalent for equivalent. Property, because each disposes of what is his own. And Bentham, because each looks only to his own advantage. The only force bringing them together and putting them into relation with one another, is the selfishness, the gain and the private interest of each.

(Marx, 1976, p280)

Marx is describing a phenomenal world where appearances seem to confirm theoretical principles even though they do not conform to the rest of social existence. What Marx is arguing is that the the level of reality in the sphere of exchange is one which accords with an ideological conception of the social whole and which if seen as universal is capable of obscuring the reality of social life. In other words, Marx argues, the capitalist mode of production spontaneously gives rise to ideologies that perpetuate it by according with the reality of some social situations. There is a problem with this form of analysis in that it presumes that there is only one way of perceiving the movement of capitalism. As Ranciere has noted, the agent of production once placed within certain situations will only perceive reality in a certain way, purely by virtue of the position he or she occupies. In other words, the appearances of commodity fetishism will only admit to a single interpretation.

Equally, the concept of false consciousness is one when used in a mechanical way can result in a position where the ruling classes' control over the means of cultural production ensures their complete control over an otherwise divided society. It has also allowed the notion to grow that the actual understandings of people are unimportant, incorrect and as such are not "real". However, this is not to say that when treated as part of a more general theory of ideology ideas such as commodity fetishism and false consciousness are not useful concepts. As to the form that this theory would take, it would be the argument of this work that we must start from Marx's concept of practice and see ideology as shaping, and shaped by, human subjects. This involves, as we have seen above, the combination of a philosophy of consciousness with a materialist theory of determination. This allows for a subject to be involved in the principle practices of class divided production and to be affected accordingly by its contradictions. In this way, the responses at the level of consciousness to the effects of the structure are not pre-determined nor epiphenomenal.

In Marx, the combination of these two elements in a notion of the active subject who is placed within historically concrete situations which marks his early work, is the first indication of how a materialist conception of ideology could work. Of course, it is only partial and undeveloped but it does mark a starting point for a Marxist analysis of ideology and is certainly different from the starting points of the discourse theorists.

The concept of ideology after Marx

After the death of Marx, the question of ideology and its status within theory became more developed. The unavailability until the 1930's of "The German Ideology", and the collapsing of Marx's critical concept of ideology into a general term for the area of consciousness meant that the use of the concept changed in emphasis. Larrain (1983) points out that after the death of Marx there was a slow but consistent shift in the use of the term; from a negative critical position to a positive neutral one. Though not deliberate, the work of Plekhanov, Labriola, Kautsky, and Bernstein led to an acceptance that ideology was equivalent to the whole sphere of ideas. So much so, that no one challenged Lenin's eventual coining of the term "socialist ideology".

The fact that a term comes to mean something different from what it originally meant does not make the new meaning necessarily invalid, but in using a positive conception of ideology the term must now account for all social consciousness and not just those ideas which distort the real nature of the world. This brings into our discussion the whole arena of base- superstructure relationships and ideology as a level of social structure. Abercrombie (1980) in examining this conceptual shift talks of a move from class-theoretical explanation to that of mode-theoretical explanation. For him, both of these explanations are heavily functionalist but mode-theoretical explanations must remove completely any question of subjectivity if they are to be consistent.

The discussion of the later Marxists will repeatedly show how an unacknowledged positive conception of ideology marks their work, even though it is used simultaneously with the negative concept.

Georg Lukacs

From this discussion of Marx's approach to ideology and consciousness, what is apparent is that Marx's notion of ideology is one that is based on human activity; insofar that it is within Man's practical relationship with nature (in producing and reproducing his existence) that the most important forms of consciousness occur. Whilst it is true that the productive process is the most important determinant in creating consciousness, it also needs to be stated that this is not an undifferentiated process. What mediates between this practical relationship and the ideas produced by it is firstly the fact that production takes place under specific social relations such as capitalism; and secondly that the dominant intellectual ideas in any society are often those that operate in the interests of the class in power. This means that a true consciousness of reality may not correspond with actual consciousness thus creating, in certain cases, ideology. And it is this difference that identifies the work of Georg Lukacs. Lukacs referred to these two aspects of understanding of the social world, as "ascribed consciousness" and "psychological consciousness"[3]. The first refers to the consciousness appropriate to a classes" objective economic interests[4] over time, whilst the latter explains the current level of awareness of a class. In bourgeois society, the proletariat has a psychological consciousness up to the point where it becomes socialist through the revolutionary process, or until it adopts a socialist consciousness in line with its objective interests. In determining the precise form that this psychological consciousness takes the crucial concept for Lukacs is reification. By this he is essentially referring to Marx's concept of commodity fetishism. As stated above this is where the phenomenal forms of the economy (ie, the fairness of exchange, the "hidden hand" of market forces, etc.) present themselves as natural relations ensuring that the real relations are hidden to human beings. In this way the capitalist system reproduces itself. However, the reification of capitalism does not have the same effects on all classes. This "naturalism" of capitalism operates in the interests of the capitalist class and because this classes" consciousness accords with the reified reality of capitalism, the bourgeoise within such a society, according to Lukacs, operates at the level of its ascribed consciousness rather than having a psychological consciousness of its position.

As Stedman Jones (1977) notes, while there are similarities between Lukacs' description of class consciousness and Weber's concept of the "ideal type", and although it is true that Weber did influence his early intellectual development, what separates Lukacs from Weber is that, for Lukacs, class consciousness is something that will occur in reality and accordingly has a role to play in the dialectical development of History; whereas for Weber the use of the "ideal type" is as an interpretive tool for understanding social phenomena. The distinction is important as it is the role of consciousness in "History" that interests Lukacs and which situates all his ideas.

Stated simply, History is for Lukacs the progression of economic-ideological "totalities", each expressive of the life conditions of successive class subjects which are moving in a particular direction - towards freedom. Stedman Jones points out: "Each class subject possesses a conception of the world which dominates and totally permeates the historical totality which it inhabits"(p37). As pointed out above, ideology therefore has the function of expressing a truth about society from the position of a particular class. Moreover, as the proletariat is by definition a universal class in that it cannot exploit any other group once it comes to power, then it must express the truth about society as it alone can see it as a totality. In other words, they are, to use Lukacs' borrowed Hegelian term, "the identical subject and object of history".

Viewed in this light the proletariat is both falsely conscious and potentially fully conscious. However Lukacs never provides a mechanism for one to lead to another, other than that of an economic collapse. This failure, it can be argued, results from the way in which Lukacs envisaged the role of his theories and of the proletariat. He sees in them the salvation of the German idealist philosophical tradition, in which he participated in as a member of the "Heidelburg school" alongside Weber and other notable neo-Kantians. Hence the importance from his perspective of establishing the working class as the "identical subject-object of history". Stedman-Jones argues that it is this idealism that provides the real impetus for Lukacs' ideas as well as the basis for his difficulties. In trying to, as Lukacs agrees, "out Hegel, Hegel" (Lukacs, 1971, pxxiii) Lukacs retreats into a variety of Kantianism stressing the transendental importance of ideas. For while on the one hand reification prevents the working class seeing their true interests, it is only a revolution of consciousness that can push them to the point of understanding their true position on the other. As Lukacs writes in "History and Class Consciousness":

> When the worker knows himself as a commodity, his knowledge is practical. That is to say, this knowledge brings about an objective structural change in the object of knowledge.
> (Lukacs, 1971, p169)

Thus ideas can be said to determine reality. There are also other difficulties associated with Lukacs' "idealistic" approach to the question of ideology. One of the most important is his failure to adequately discuss the contradictory nature of consciousness. He constantly talks about the reified consciousness of the proletariat or the class ideology of the proletariat (Marxism) but does not have a great deal to say about the gradations in between. In many respects this replicates Lenin's schema in "What is to be done?", where there is an absolute dichotomy between bourgeois ideology and socialist consciousness. While Lenin still had room for the various different aspects of "contaminated" ideology such as trade union consciousness and reformist consciousness (eventually discarding his underplaying of class struggle in creating political consciousness (see Molyneaux, 1978)), Lukacs was forced to keep his absolute categories because of their philosophical importance. Thus there is a necessary polarisation between the pure class ideologies of "fundamental" classes and any form of actual consciousness that did not reach these high standards. As McCarney points out when discussing this aspect of Lukacs' work:

> If one assumes that ideologies serve class interests and that the interests of classes are irreconcilably opposed. There is a difficulty in seeing how there can be any contaminated, in the sense of "compound" or syncretic ideologies. It becomes impossible for class ideologies to incorporate significant elements from the ideology of other classes without losing their identity.
> (McCarney, 1980, p52)

Lukacs' philosophy puts severe limitations on the usefulness of his conception of ideology. Even if it is accepted, as McCarney later points out, that this underplays the distinction between psychological consciousness and ascribed consciousness and that ideology is merely the class level of understanding; it is still the fact that all we really have is a philosophy.

On the positive side, in spite of much of Lukacs' work being problematic in its attachment to German idealism, it incorporates many concepts and themes that are important to retain. Concepts that later thinkers have tried to bury. The most obvious is his clear commitment to Marxism as a revolutionary practice and to the importance of class consciousness within it. His attachment to the idea of false consciousness is also valuable. Yet this is one idea that Lukacs has been particularly, but wrongly, attacked for holding. As Larrain (1983) points out many of the criticisms of Lukacs' work stem from the falsely ascribed notion that

183

he saw all ideology as false consciousness. Here the problem is the conflation of positive and negative conceptions of ideology in the minds of those criticizing him. As noted above, Lukacs does not believe that bourgeois class consciousness is false because it is ideological, but because the bourgeois class position is structurally limited. In this way, Lukacs' analysis of false consciousness is not a theory of ideology itself, but is a theory of the nature of bourgeois ideology.

Critics of Lukacs, such as McDonough (1977), use ideology in its negative sense and ignore his use of it as a positive conception. As a result the wrongly conclude that Lukacs saw all ideology as false consciousness. Similarly, the criticism made by Hirst (1979) that it is as ludicrous to describe any form of consciousness as false "as it is to describe a black pudding as false" both distorts and misses the point. As Eagleton (1991) points out it confuses "false" as in "untrue" with "false" as in "unreal" and subsequently confuses epistemological questions with ontological ones. Furthermore, it is not the case that because the consciousness of a group, or of an individual, is labelled false it is of no account. Most of what occurs in society is as the result of such consciousness and most thinkers using the term are aware of this and do not disregard such activity.

Another strength that Lukacs possesses compared with later "structuralist" readings of ideology, is his acknowledgement in his later work "Lenin"(1973) that ideology (in its positive form) and social consciousness are inextricably linked. In other words that the ideas in peoples" heads have to be seen in relation to a concept of "objective interests" and that these form the bases for action. In this he is following Marx who argued in his "Theses on Feuerbach":"That human subjects are not merely contemplative, they are also involved in practice and especially in revolutionary practice" (Marx, in Engels, 1978, p66) and also the Bolshevik tradition. Consequently, although Lukacs fails to theorise ideology and consciousness adequately, what he does do is raise the question of how class consciousness comes about within the context of bourgeois ideology. It is possible to develop out of these ideas notions whereby limited forms of class consciousness can develop from the failure of bourgeois ideology to explain the totality of capitalism. This is especially evident in those aspects of social life where conflict is a day to-day- reality. This aspect will be elucidated later.

Louis Althusser

The importance of the work of the French philosopher Louis Althusser[5] cannot be overemphasised. Indeed much of the contemporary debate about the nature of ideology derives from the interest generated by his work. His work has a double importance for this research in that it represents the most significant attempt to "marry" together Marxism with structuralism and has been the starting point for what Sumner (1980) called the structuralist "avant garde" within Marxism.

In presenting a structuralist or "theoretical anti-humanist" conception of Marxism, Althusser had first to settle accounts with the ideas of his predecessors - most notably the ideas of Lukacs. In opposition to him, Althusser challenged the role of active human agency in Marxist theory. Althusser's major objection to what he termed Lukacs' historicist reading of Marx was the role it gave to consciousness and subjectivity in the processes of History. In its place Althusser asserted the primacy of structure in determining the activity of human individuals. In much the same way that Levi-Strauss saw primitive societies directed by the form of mythology or totemism they adopted, Althusser argued that it was not enough to say that human agents act within the confines of social structures. instead he states that humans are, in essence, supports to those structures. It is beyond the scope of this work to describe how Althusser conceived of the nature of social structure, but within his concept of structures-in-dominance ideology is given a whole level of its own complete with its own relative autonomy (this is implicit in his distinction between ideology in general and particular ideologies). In "For Marx" Althusser uses the term ideology in the most positive sense imaginable, consigning to it all mental products. It is simultaneously concerned with both the realm of consciousness and with the realm of deception. Ideology exists not only to equip the mode of production with its complement of labourers but also to perpetuate the inequalities of a class system by systematically covering up contradictions. It is this that leads Althusser to state that ideology is a set of lived false relationships that people have to their real conditions of existence:

> In ideology men do indeed express, not the relation between them and their conditions of existence but the way they live the relation between than and their condition of existence: thus pre-supposes both a real relation and an "imaginary" lived relation.
> (Althusser, 1977, p233)

Althusser can argue from this that ideology has a structural basis independent of the wills of men. At one stroke dispensing with the need for concepts such as false consciousness. As we have seen, Abercrombie (1980) described this as a move from a class theoretical position to a mode theoretical one which removes the importance of class interests. It also diminishes the importance of ideas and consciousness. To quote Althusser once again:

> Ideology is indeed a system of representations, but in the majority of cases, these representations have nothing to do with "consciousness", they are usually images and occasionally concepts, but it is above all as structures that they impose on the vast majority of men, not via their "consciousness".
> (Althusser, 1977, p233)

A radical division between Althusser's conception and previous Marxist views becomes manifest. This becomes even more apparent when we look at the precise way Althusser sees the operation of ideological structures. For him human subjects are interpellated or "hailed" by ideology in much the same way a passenger hails a taxi. Individuals have no independent role to play in all of this and are incapable of acting outside of the determination of ideology. Moreover, interpellation is a process that is invested by Althusser with the ability to create "individuals".

> The practico-social function specific to ideology is to constitute concrete individuals as subjects to transform individuals into subjects. Indeed it is by its concrete functioning in the material rituals of everyday life that every individual recognises himself as a "subject". This recognition of being a subject (with such characteristics as uniqueness, freedom, etc.), thus recognition of what appears to be an obvious and natural fact is in fact an ideological recognition of an obviousness imposed by ideology. One recognises oneself as a subject only in the practice of concrete ideological rituals inscribed in ideological apparatuses.
> (McLennan, Molina, Peters, 1977, p96)

The process of interpellation operates through the medium of social institutions in order to have the material effects described above. These institutions - ideological state apparatuses (ISA's) are brought into being by the structures of the mode of production itself, whilst at the same time they serve the interests of the dominant class. Althusser numbers among them: the schools; the church; the trade unions and most other large institutions that exist in modern society.

However, even in terms of Althusser's own premises there has been criticism. Perry Anderson (1977) points out that it is impossible for institutions as varied as the church, schools or the mass media to be regarded as being part of the state without the notion of the specificity of the state being destroyed; and in so doing breaking down any distinction between civil society and the repressive role of the state. Consequently, the focus for ideological mediation through institutions is lost.

If there can be one major criticism of Althusser's position it is that there is little room for Marxist politics. If all thought is ideological and cohesive, where do Communists come from? As Larrain suggests:

> If the general function of ideology is to secure everyone's adhesion to the system and if the particular "overdetermined" function of ideology is to secure the domination of the ruling class, how can this very ideology be the vehicle of protest? If ideology is said to "interpellate" individuals and to "constitute" them as "subjects" obedient to the system, how can they, through an ideological tendency, become critical of the system?
> (Larrain, 1983, p93)[6]

In evaluating the usefulness of the Althusserian project we become aware once again of the fact that the very attractiveness of structuralism is what creates its ultimate weakness as far as the question of ideology is concerned; namely its over emphasis on structure to the detriment of human agency.

Therborn (1980) in his "The Power of Ideology, the Ideology of Power", attempts to overcome thus deficiency by postulating the idea of classes each being differentially interpellated within ideology in accordance with their social positions, class struggle occurs in this schema through the medium of class alter ideologies. As he explains:

> The crucial aspect of the alter-ideology is in the case of the exploiting classes, the rationale for their domination of other classes. In the case of exploited classes, it is the basis for their resistance to the exploiters.
> (Therborn, 1980, p61)

As Therborn himself admits what this does is to reduce the phenomena of class struggle to articulations of these class alter- ideologies, which it could be argued is merely another variant of idealism.

If Therborn represents an attempt to overcome the problem of subjectivity by giving an Althusserian base to it, others have decided that the problem is the question of consciousness itself and here we return to the starting point of the "New Revisionism". Namely structuralism triumphing over Marxism. The work of Coward and Ellis (1977) and Hirst (1979) represent this shift. Anxious to retain ideology as an objective level of society they saw the problems besetting Althusser as being overcome by a more rigorous structural linguistics.

Ideology as a lived practice is obviously an important conception and development of Marxist theory, and it is true that Poulantzas (1975) in his usage of the concept of juridico-political citizens uses it to great effect. However, in its form as developed by Althusser (and post-Althusserians such as Pecheaux, 1982) it is limited in the same way that structuralism is limited, in other words in its reliance on structural forms of ideology dominating social agents' understanding of reality. Thus the notion of ideology as self referential and hermetically sealed becomes a problem of epistemology and not of social analysis. "Truth" is theoretical rather than practical. In this conception there is no way out of the ideological maze as a penetration through to "reality" is precluded[7]. The acceptance of ideology as eternal, which is the consequence of this position, is too dismissive of human subjectivity. Ideologies certainly do operate by excluding areas of difficulty from their field of explanation but the dynamics of a social formation do not exclude the ideology (or ideologies) from being forced to confront them. If this was true ideology wouldn't be necessary.

A final criticism of Althusser's project is that it fails to discuss one of the most important levels of ideology, namely that of its practical operation. Ideology operates at the level of articulated ideas whose meanings are often fought over and the concept needs to be examined in this context as well. Failure to do this is to leave everything at the same abstract level as Lukacs" work. Here the worry voiced has been that if ideas are discussed as an important part of ideology then Marxist analysis would be guilty of an idealist deviation. However, as Larrain (1983) points out, this argument is predicated on the notion that if we talk about ideas we cannot be talking about material reality at the same time. This is simply not the case. As he says, forms of social consciousness can only exist if they are inscribed in social practices. He argues that in their attempt "to give consciousness an unquestionable reality, Althusser, and Hirst after him, have fallen into the trap of considering such a reality only in the form of an object, as an external materiality, not subjectively. They have avoided one kind of reductionism at the cost of falling into another, namely the reductionism of considering consciousness and ideology confronting subjects from without. It is as if the reality of social consciousness could be guaranteed only by its objectivation" (Larrain, 1983, p102). Following Larrain it is possible to talk of ideas in the context of ideology and still root them in material practices.

Antonio Gramsci

I have left the work of Antonio Gramsci until last, because rather than deal with the development of Marxist theory chronologically, what I wanted to do was to set up a number of base lines from which difficulties could be drawn and then show how Gramsci's ideas help us to understand them. So far, I have been arguing that we must understand ideology as a negative concept, that is as a process whereby reality is distorted to the benefit of a dominant class. This distortion pervades all areas of social life and is present in all institutions. Social consciousness is based on social practice, so ideology has to be constantly made and remade if it is to fulfill its role. Similarly, in all sorts of different forms, a "true" or partially true understanding of reality is always present in social practice. As a result social harmony is not automatic.

The work of Gramsci is useful to us because unlike Lukacs and Althusser he was not principally an academic. His role as leader of the Italian Communist Party in the 1920s meant that for him the problems of ideology and political consciousness were practical ones rather than just ones of an academic nature. This led him to conceive of the problem of ideology differently and to emphasise the importance of the institutional mediators of ideas and knowledge in capitalist society.

Crucial to Gramsci's project was the division he saw existing between the East and the West. In the East it was the state that was determinant in maintaining social order, whilst in the West it was civil society that performed this role. Gramsci, in making this distinction, was not denying the basic similarity in function of the state in both the East and the West. Indeed in the "Lyons Theses" (see Harman, 1984) he had clearly argued for the need to see the state as essentially a repressive force. Instead, what he wanted to show was that, because in the West there was a more developed social structure, than in the East, it allowed these societies to function with at least a minimal level of consent.

As Anderson (1977) has noted, Gramsci, when attempting to theorise the nature of the relation between state and civil society fell into a number of conceptual errors - even finding it difficult to define civil society itself. Whilst Anderson points to at least three different ways that Gramsci conceived of the relationship between the state and civil society, it is only one that need interest us. This is the one where Gramsci excludes the economy from civil society and asserts that the state is the outer ditch of defence for civil society. In the West the juridico-political elements were the main contribution to the stability of society and that as a consequence economic instability was less effective in bringing about social change than ideological factors. Anderson argues that this is the result of a fundamental misunderstanding on Gramsci's part. The role of the state in the West is not less important but more important. This is due to what he describes as the 'structural asymmetry" between the state and civil society, which results from civil society's ability only to provide ideological functions for the continuation of bourgeois power. The state can provide these at the same time as having a monopoly of legitimate violence is therefore more powerful.

> It is impossible to partition the ideological functions of bourgeoise class power between "civil society" and the state in the way Gramsci originally sought to do. The fundamental form of the western parliamentary state, the juridical sum of its citizenry - is itself the hub of the ideological apparatuses of capitalism.
> (Anderson, 1977, p29)

Anderson argues that because of this the power of ideological factors must not be overestimated. It is true that Western bourgeois democracies are dominated by culture, but as he points out they are determined by coercion.

This flaw in Gramsci's work leads him to overestimate the impact of what he describes as the "hegemonic bloc" which leads one class to dominate all others and to incorporate its world view into theirs[8]. Here Gramsci, as Harman has pointed out, is trying to make generalisations about class struggle from the rise of the bourgeoise to power under Feudalism. The rising capitalist class were only capable of developing intellectual hegemony over the aristocracy because it had the economic resources to organise it and could make alliances with previously dominant classes without contradicting their interests. For example, commodity production initially takes place within Feudal society allowing for both economic and political power to develop without challenge. The working class under capitalism can do neither of these things.

While the notion of the "hegemonic bloc" has serious limitations other ideas that are contained within this framework do have considerable application. Gramsci viewed ideology as operating at different levels. According to Larrain (1983) there are at least four - Philosophy, Religion, Commonsense, and Folklore. Philosophy is the most systematic and rigorous form of ideology, the best expression of a world view of a class. As Gramsci writes "Philosophy is intellectual order, which neither religion nor commonsense can be" (Gramsci, 1971, p325). All philosophies other than Marxism are "lacerated" by the contradictions inherent in their class origins and must therefore be viewed as false. Marxism escapes this categorisation because as a science it is aware of these contradictions and seeks actively to overcome them. This leads Gramsci to describe Marxism as "the Philosophy of Praxis".

This emphasis on activity is not accidental. It is not merely that ideology exists as a set of ideas that is important, but that these ideas are bound up in and consequently explain action. Gramsci's understanding of what he describes as Religion illustrates this. He suggest that Religion operates not just as articles of faith but is also the source of practical orientations for action. So, although Religion lacks the intellectual order and coherence of Philosophy, it does have the ability to permeate into popular culture - it allows Philosophy to be socialised. Similarly, Gramsci's notion of Commonsense is of an ideological form that is more incoherent and inarticulate than Religion, but is accordingly more pervasive among the subordinated classes. Finally, Folklore being the lowest degree of ideology is a collection of disparate elements from various world views, without much coherence.

Built into all of Gramsci's conceptions of ideology is that as they become more effective their ideological clarity becomes more fragmented. Because of this, it is to the notion of "Commonsense" that I want to pay particular attention. As Anderson (1980) points out, despite its connotation in English, Commonsense is ordinarily very far removed from the real needs and interests of the masses of ordinary people who hold it. Thought that does achieve this is referred to by Gramsci as "goodsense."

Commonsense has the advantage that it is never simply identical with ruling class ideology. This ideology at best "only limits the original thought, of the popular masses in a negative direction" (Adamson, 1980, p150). Commonsense argues Gramsci must be understood as a series of stratified deposits of previous philosophies;

It contains stone age elements, and principles of a more advanced science, prejudices from all phases of history at the local level and

191

> intuitions of a future philosophy which will be that of a human
> race united the world over.
> (Gramsci, 1971, p324)

Because of this Gramsci's notion of Commonsense is not one that is rigid and immobile, but one that is continually "transforming itself, enriching itself, with scientific ideas that have entered ordinary life."(Gramsci, 1971, p326) Adamson argues that it this ability that ensures that Commonsense is more likely to incorporate philosophical challenges as new sedimentation within an ever shifting whole, than it is to be exposed and overthrown. However, Adamson goes on to argue that "intractability is compounded by the embeddedness of Commonsense within language itself" (Adamson, 1980, p150) and thus makes escape from ideology difficult.

> For Gramsci, an historically organic ideology, - as opposed to the
> idiosyncratic ruminations of a particular individual - is not a
> naked conceptual scheme but a class weltanshauung clothed in the
> language, "mores", and ways of life of a particular culture. Like
> all ideologies, Commonsense may have "true" elements but is
> never a confirmation of truth. Its relation to truth is wholly
> subordinate to its function as the cement smoothing relations
> between state and civil society.
> (Adamson, 1980, p151)

The discussion of Gramsci's work, so far, has concentrated on the cultural mediations of ideological forms which can lead to an idealist reading of his work. However, Gramsci did see the need for ideology to be rooted in the processes of everyday life. Gramsci's way of connecting this was through the medium of class struggle itself. An important point for Gramsci was that ideologies do vary in their social roles, some are merely systems of mystification, whilst others are the medium through which members of classes become aware of conflicts and fight them out. The transformation from one to another is brought about by a series of negations - negations which expose and repudiate the "prevailing Commonsense." However, this transformation does not come about by purely intellectual activity alone, but is developed by the contradictory nature of class society and the material forms that are based upon it; and in so doing goes in part to answer Adamsons belief in the intractability of Commonsense.

192

What Gramsci is discussing is the gap that exists between a hegemonic ideology coming through what ever form and a subordinates class activity:

> ...is it not often the case that there is a contradiction between ones intellectual affirmation and ones mode of conduct? Which then is the real conception of the world: that logically affirmed as an intellectual act? Or that which emerges from the real activity of each man, which is implicit in his behaviour.
> (Gramsci, quoted in Femia, 1981, p43)

As Femia (1981) elaborates what Gramsci is pointing to is the distinction between "true" and "false" consciousness.

> ...this contrast between thought and action ...cannot but be the expression of profounder contrasts of a social historical order. It signifies that the relevant social group (the working class) has its own conception of the world even if only embryonic, a conception which manifests itself in action, but occasionally, by fits and starts - when that is the group is acting as an organic totality. But this same group has for reasons of submission and intellectual subordination adopted a conception which is not its own but is borrowed from another group.
> (Gramsci, quoted in Femia, 1981, p43)

Thus out of the notion of Commonsense develops the important idea of dual consciousness:

> The Active man-in-the-mass has a practical activity, but has no theoretical consciousness of this activity. One might almost say that he has two theoretical consciousnesses (or one contradictory consciousness) one which is implicit in his activity and which truly unites him with all his fellow workers in the practical transformation of reality; and one superficially explicit or verbal which he has inherited from the past and partially accepted.
> (Gramsci, 1971, p333)

Dual consciousness as a concept goes some way towards overcoming the dualism outlined earlier in the discussion on Marx. By conceiving ideology as a contradictory form we can see its determination by the ideological domination of a ruling class A determination which simultaneously involves the active conscious response of the subordinated class in an albeit fragmented form.

A criticism of the Gramscian formulation is that it treats the worker's involvement in the productive process too unproblematically. It sees the very fact that there are contradictions within the capitalist mode of production as being sufficient to produce a class conscious working class, only prevented from the realisation of its true position by the effect of bourgeois hegemony. This same fault has been noted with Lukacs' formulations and originates from an idealist philosophical background being superimposed upon Marxism, andproduces a faith in the inevitable collapse of capitalism and in the power of consciousness. Here, it is useful to bring back Althusser's notion of ideology as "lived practice." This, Therborn (1980) achieves when writing about what he calls the proletarian alter-ideology. For Therborn, the working class does not merely accept a dominant ideology, but generates its own, under conditions that are influenced by capitalist social relations. What predominates in capitalist society is the buying and selling of labour power on the market. This causes a split in working class consciousness:

> On the one hand they are individuals market agents, free and equal in relation to the purchasers of labour power. On the other hand, they also constitute a separate class (in the logical sense) of market agents having only a very special commodity to trade, their labour power, which is an inseparable part of human capacity. Inherent in this situation seems to be resistance to the total conversion of labour power into a commodity: an assertion of the working person with rights to employment, adequate subsistence and some degree of security counterposed to the commodity rationality of the market and of capital accumulation.
> (Therborn, 1980, p62-63)

For Therborn the basis for dual consciousness lies in both the market rationality of the sale of wage labour and in attempts to resist this incorporation - which can only come at the expense of those selling their labour. Therborn points out that the second part of this dualism, that of the response, does not create automatic class consciousness, instead it creates a proletarian stress on collectivity and solidarity as opposed to competitive individualism - but this stress is as much a competitive collectivism as it is socialist - for it is still bounded by the market. This conception in many ways frees the analysis of dual consciousness from an automatic equation between experience and class domination. It is something that Perry Anderson (1980) in his discussion of E.P.

Thompson's "The Making of the English Working Class" has sought to bring out. He argues that there is a need to make a distinction between the experience that people have of their everyday lives and the experience that leads them to come to conclusions. Talking of the second form he writes: "Here, experience itself remains an objective sector of "social being" which is than processed or handled by the subject to yield a particular "social consciousness". The possibility of different ways of different ways of "handling" the same experience is epistemologically secured"(Anderson, 1980, pp28- 29).

What this then allows is a theory of "dual consciousness" that starts from a base in human practical activity (in other words, work), which allows practice to simultaneously produce a "market" ideology. This corresponds with Poulantzas' (1980) notion of the Juridico-political individual, and is capable of forming the basis of resistance to incorporation into the market. Similarly, at the cultural level, ideas can contain both hegemonic and subversive elements - their precise articulation dependent on the balance of forces outside the ideological arena.

In conclusion what has been argued here is that an important aspect of a Marxist theory of ideology is seeing the dialectical nature of the relation between ideas and social forms. Moreover, it must also be based, at least to some extent, on the conscious activity of those who are held under its sway. Therefore I would argue that Gramsci's notion of "dual consciousness" offers the most comprehensive framework for understanding the working of ideology.

Notes

1. For an accessible account of Hegel's philosophy see Singer (1983).

2. See: Althussser (1971, 1979), Althusser and Balibar (1979), Draper (1975), Hook (1965).

3. Apart from Lukacs" own "History and Class Consciousness" (1971) which contains the essays "Class Consciousness" and "Reification and the Consciousness of the Proletariat" other useful works on the work of Lukacs are Arato (1972), Stedman-Jones (1977), Arato and Breines (1979), Lowy (1979) and Larrain (1983).

4. Within Marxist theory there is a large debate on what constitute "objective economic interests" or even whether they even exist (see Kitching, 1983). But, for the purposes of this research we shall accept a

definition of class interests being those in which the demands of a particular mode of production lead to irreconcilable contradiction between the interests of contending social classes. Thus the need for profit in capitalism comes into conflict with the need of the labourer to sell labour power at its highest price. The objective interest of the worker is thus to diminish the power of the employing class. Furthermore, the cyclical economic movement of booms and slumps means that the worker, in order to avoid these ravages has an interest in abolishing capitalism as a system. However, Wright (1985) contends that the notion of "true interests" is linked to the kinds of preference that people make to increase their freedom and autonomy. "Insofar as the actual capacity that individuals have to make choices and act upon them - their real freedom - is shaped systematically by their position within the class structure, they have objective class interests based on this real interest in freedom. To the extent that the conscious preferences of people lead them to make choices which reduce that capacity or block its expansion, then, I would say, they are acting against their "true" or "objective" class interests" (Wright, 1985, p249).

5. Most of what Althusser has had to say has not come in the form of books, but rather in the form of numerous essays contained in the following collections. "Reading Capital"(with Etiene Balibar) (1979), "For Marx" (1979),and "Lenin and Philosophy"(1979).

6. Lovell (1980) has also developed a sustained critique of Althusser along these lines.

7. A suitable starting point for the theorists of "post-moderism" to start from, given their widespread insistence on the death of grand narratives and the essential "ironic" quality of social understanding.

8. This is probably what leads many Eurocommunist readings of Gramsci to develop in the direction that they do. See Buci-Glucksman (1980), Showstack-Sassoon (1982) etc .

10 Ideology 3: The duality of structure?

Marxist theory is not the only intellectual system where the question of dual consciousness is raised. The idea is also important to the more recent work of the sociologist Anthony Giddens. While drawing on the work of Marx and calling himself a socialist (1982a), his work is radically different from that of the Marxists discussed. For this reason alone it is worth looking at. A more important reason however, is that in discussing the relationship between agency and structure Giddens brings to light important considerations that help us to broaden our understanding of the concept of dual consciousness.

This section will therefore begin by discussing Giddens' concept of "the duality of structure" in general terms before turning to a more specific discussion of the nature and development of working class consciousness in developed capitalist societies.

Giddens (1979) sees his argument for "the duality of structure" as "connecting a motion of human action with structural explanation in social analysis". This is by no means an easy task as Dallmayr (1982) has pointed out:

Giddens has seen himself faced with a momentous challenge: the challenge of incorporating the lessons of ontology and post structuralism without abandoning concern with the "knowledgability" and accountability of actors; more ambitiously phrased: the task of moving beyond subjectivist metaphysics without relinquishing some of its insights, and especially without lapsing into objectivism and determinism.

(Dallmayr, 1982, p19)

At a philosophical level what Giddens is attempting to do is develop the "human conduct as the product of intentional action" traditions of hermeneutics and post-Wittgensteinian analytical philosophy, into an account capable of coping with conceptions of structural explanation and social causation. Immediately, it will be apparent that Giddens is wrestling with the same problem that faced Marx. How to tread the fine line between voluntarism and determinism without subordinating one to the other.

Giddens wants to argue that "Action" and "Structure" which are usually presented as antimonies in social thought, do in fact presuppose one another - they exist and can only exist as a dialectical relationship . As Giddens writes in reply to one of his critics.

All social life is inherently creative, in the sense that it is carried in and through the knowledgeable activities engaged in by agents in the course of their day-to-day lives. Social systems do not have form or continuity across time and space, because they are programmed to do so by some mysterious set of causal forces propelling individuals along pre- prepared pathways. On the other hand, situated actors do not create most of what they do in the sense of inventing it, ex nihilo. Quite to the contrary, they act in social contexts whose modes of organisation precede their existence in time, and spread out laterally in space.

(Giddens, 1985, p170)

The idea of the "duality of structure" operates under the more inclusive concept of structuration - the term being borrowed from Derrida and referring to the structuring of structures themselves.

The concept of structuration involves that of the duality of structure, which relates to the fundamentally recursive character of social life, and expresses the mutual dependence of structure and agency. By the duality of structure I mean that the stuctural properties of social systems are both the medium and the outcome of the practices that constitute those systems.

(Giddens, 1979, p69)

According to Giddens, the theory of structuration means that the same structural characteristics participate in the subject (actor) as in the object (society). Consequently, "structure forms "personality" and society simultaneously" (Giddens, 1979, p70)) both being part of the same movement. Social structures enter the scene then as "the unacknowledged conditions and unanticipated consequences" of human conduct. Giddens distinguishes sharply between these structures and social systems, the latter referring to the persistences in time and space of human collectivities.

Every social system possesses a set of "structural principles" which are the structural elements that are most deeply embedded in the space-time dimensions of social systems and which govern the basic institutional alignments of a society. In this way Giddens is able to describe three main components of structure: signification, domination, and legitimation, Domination refers to the imbalance of utilisable resources in power relations, while legitimation describes the nature of the non-coercive forms giving rise to claims to resources and signification is the communication and rationisation of human actions by means of interpretative schemes. Structural principles typically involve social contradictions, so that whilst they operate in terms of one another they at the same time contravene one another. As Callinicos (1985c) points out the strength of this outlook is its anti- functionalism. This is illustrated in the way that Giddens is aware that not only do social practices have functional attributes but that they also contain contradictions. Similarly, at a theoretical level, structuration does not accept that the existence of structures in itself explains the persistence of social systems.

The theory, while bringing into interpretative understanding notions of structure and determination, must be understood in the context that its force comes from putting human action at its centre:

> Although structure shapes the conduct of human agents, it is only through that conduct that it itself possesses any effectivity, and it may itself be modified by the activity of which it is the unacknowledged condition and unanticipated consequence.
>
> (Callinicos, 1985c, p137)

It is this aspect of Giddens' ideas that I will return to shortly because in many ways it is at the centre of criticisms of his work, but first I want to explore in some more depth his development of the processes whereby human activity takes place. For Giddens, Action or Agency refers to a continuous flow of conduct involving intentionality as process as well as reflexive monitoring of conduct. As he explains; intentionality is a routine feature of human conduct and does not imply that actors have definite goals consciously held in mind during the course of their activity "that the latter is unusual in fact, is indicated in ordinary English usage, by the distinction between meaning or intending to do something and doing something "purposefully" the latter implying an uncommon degree of mental application given to the pursuit of an aim"(Giddens, 1979, p56).

That social actors have more than intentionality is shown by Giddens' use of the notion of "reflexive monitoring". Here not only have individuals the ability to do things but they are also able to provide an understanding of why they do or want to do certain things.

> The reflexive monitoring of behavior operates against the background of the rationalisation of action - by which I mean the capabilities of human agents to "explain" why they act as they do by giving reasons for their conduct - and in the more "inclusive" context of practical consciousness[1].
>
> (Giddens, 1979, p57)

The usefulness of this approach is demonstrated in Giddens comments about Braverman's work on the labour process, here he introduces into his notion of action the concepts of power and domination which he feels are "logically, and not just contingently, associated with the concepts of action and structure" (Giddens, 1982c, p29). What follows, therefore, is that in all situations there must exist a "dialectic of control" between those with power and those affected by it. The crucial term to remember here is dialectic. Giddens explains in the following terms:

> Power relations in social systems can be regarded as relations of autonomy and dependence; but no matter how imbalanced they may be in termsof power, actors in subordinate positions are never wholly dependent, and are often very adept at converting whatever resources they possess into some degree of control over the conditions of reproduction of the system. In all social systems there is a dialectic of control, such that there are, normally continually shifting balances of resources, altering the overall distribution of power.
>
> (Giddens, 1982c, p32)

It is this dualism in Giddens' work that must lead back to Marxist analysis. This is because one of the consequences of seeing domination and power as separate from economics is that there is now no necessity for conflict to be placed at the heart of economic relations. Instead, they are formally distinct from one another. Even within Giddens' notion of domination there is no necessary connection.

Thus Giddens is drawn to criticise Braverman on the grounds that he perceives the processes of capitalist domination in the workplace as operating in one direction only. The question of whether this may be an exaggeration of Braverman's work is not important. What is important is that Giddens, using his concept of the knowledgability of human actors, is able to see social processes in a much more dynamic form than is usual in most social analysis. As he writes "what is lacking (in Braverman) is an adequate discussion of the reactions of workers, as themselves knowledgeable and capable agents to the technical division of labour and to Taylorism" (Giddens, 1982c, p40).

Giddens, in a similar way to Mann (1973) goes on to point out that it is important not to sever the "subjective" from the "objective" components of class; that it is possible to equate class consciousness only with Marx's notion of class "for itself" and consequently to ignore the actual consciousness of class members by concentrating purely on the "objective" features of class.

All class relations obviously involve the conscious activity of human agents. But this is different from groups of individuals being conscious of being members of the same class, of having common class interests, and so on. It is quite possible to conceive of circumstances in which individuals are not only cognisant of being in a common class situation, but where they may actively deny the existence of classes - and where their attitudes and ideas can nevertheless be explained in terms of class relationships.

(Giddens, 1982c, p40)

However, there is a price to be paid for being able to ground social theory so strongly in the actual practices and understandings of human subjects. This price, argues Callinicos, is the tendency to collapse structure into agency.

The way in which Giddens conceptualises structure means that it can only function as a secondary aspect of social practice, subject to the creative interventions of "knowledgeable human agents". The result, as Habermas points out is "an anthropomorphic concept of society" in which the subject rules supreme, producing society as labour produces use value. Far from overcoming the dualism of agency and structure, Giddens is stuck firmly at the pole of agency. The much invoked 'duality of structure" amounts to little more than a substitution of two letters - a verbal change.

(Callinicos, 1985c, p155)

This charge wouldn't be so serious if it wasn't for the consequences that it entails. These originate in the way in which the concept of structuration is seen by Giddens as essential part of his whole project to create a non-functionalist variety of social analysis. This desire to have non-functionalist forms of explanation does not just cover the more obvious forms of Parsonian and Althusserian thought but all functional explanations (Giddens, 1982a, pp18-19). Indeed as Cohen (1987) points out Giddens' theory of structuration requires a rejection of the principle of uniformity which underlies the existence of trans-historical regularities. Thus arguments ranging from the necessity of capitalism to maintain a reserve army of labour to the function of state policies in optimising capital accumulation, are regarded as illegitimate.

What this then allows him to do is to make a split between the economic basis of a society and its social forms. Class is not defined in terms of surplus extraction as in the Marxist model but in terms of how the surplus is extracted. That is whether it is done through authoritative means (by force or power) or by direct control over the means of production. In Feudalism the fact that the ruling groups appropriate resources from the peasantry by force means that the real division in these societies, though still resulting in classes is the structure of authoritative domination.

Marxist analysis on the other hand would argue that the domination of the feudal rulers resulted essentially from their economic position in controlling the means of production and not vice versa. However, in making the split in the interests of non- functionalism, Giddens is now in the position, argues Wright (1983), of putting forward the thesis that the social organisation of authoritative resources and their development and transformation is autonomous from allocative resources; that in fact there are two autonomous structures operating within societies with no general principles governing their interconnection: namely power and production. What started out as favouring the side of agency in social analysis quickly moves to stopping any analysis of the real conditions under which people act, and it is because we need to found our understanding of social consciousness in the reality of the social world that Giddens' overall project fails.

The Marxist claim that the concept of class combines the relations of economic exploitation and authoritative domination is implicitly a rejection of the claim that these have genuinely autonomous logics of

202

development; Giddens restriction of class to relations of domination with respect to allocative resources affirms his view that allocative and authoritative domination are autonomous processes.

(Wright, 1983, p32)

It is this dualism in Giddens' work that must lead us back to Marxist analysis because one of the consequences of seeing domination and power as separate from economics is for conflict to be at the heart of economic relations as these are separate, (even within domination there is no necessary conflict - it is entirely contingent). Given that Giddens also disputes that there is any historical tendency for the forces of production to develop (in fact he rejects any notion of "evolutionary" thought preferring to see modern industrial capitalism as a unique form of social organisation), what is left with in terms of social analysis is an explanation based on a rationalised form of alienation.

The more a worker comes close to being an "appendage of a machine", the more he or she ceases to be a human agent..... precisely because they are not machine, wherever they can do so, human actors devise ways of avoiding being treated as such.

(Giddens, 1982c pp44-45)

Marxism and discourse theory

If, the strength of Giddens' position lies in its acceptance of the importance of agency and human interaction with structure, then it is not enough to merely criticise it - an alternative must be provided. The elements for such an alternative have been provided by Gramsci and his notion of dual consciousness, but, it is obvious that this does not go far enough. While his concept is grounded in the practical activity of human beings, it is still true to say that he provides no basis for how consciousness becomes such. Here, the ideas of structuralism through the medium of discourse theory seem to present a superior methodology. This, in turn, downplays the importance of practical activity and leads back, ultimately, to an idealist understanding of ideology.

It is one thing to be aware of the faults of a theoretical position, it is another to be able to find an equally useful substitute. In the case of structuralist influenced theories the problem is the traditional Marxist axiom that classes are primarily objective formations, defined by social relationships of exploitation that secure the extraction of surplus labour from the immediate producers. This, quite logically, means accepting an extra-discursive starting point for discourse. On the other hand, it also means accepting the problem of reductionism. Even accepting our understanding of consciousness as an essentially practical activity does not easily get us out of this difficulty. As Marshall (1983) has argued, the various attempts (Marxist and non-Marxist) to see consciousness from the point of view of the constitutive aspects of actors existences have all failed, because, as he writes:

> While all talk has been of grounding it in the experiences and practices of every day life, of locating its social origins firmly in the immediate or distant milieux of social and cultural life, often it has been located in this manner at the front door only to slip out again, spirit like, at the back.
>
> (Marshall, 1983, p280)

What is at fault, argues Marshall, is that class consciousness becomes detached from class experience "except as a spiritual reflection of it" (Marshall, 1983, p280), so that certain structural features relating to social class membership such as the nature of work situations, occupational communities etc. automatically generate an awareness of the world. The result claims Marshall is that consciousness become "something akin to a knap-sack carried around on one's back - or in this case, one's head, - and dipped into when the occasion demanded" (Marshall, 1983, p281).

It is possible to divide many of the contemporary theorists of class consciousness into two groups; those believing in class instrumentalism and those that argue working class is essentially ambivalent. But when it comes down to it, what is found is that both tendencies lose the notion of the subject in order to concentrate on either stating the obvious about workers attempting to maximise rewards in a capitalist market situation; or alternatively, being completely overwhelmed by the complexity and seeming irrationality of ideas held by social actors.

The solution as far as Marshall is concerned, and as I have argued earlier, is to link up the notion of social consciousness with that of social action. This can only be done by realising that consciousness is generated in, and changed by, social action. To do this it is necessary to start our analysis from the position that class is generated by an antagonism which originates in the forms of production in any given society. This antagonism can be seen as an objective reality which brings about class struggle between dominant and dominated classes. While dominant classes will have social and political forms to ensure their rule (as well as structures thrown up by the mode of production itself), the very fact that there exists an antagonistic relationship between the classes must mean that members of dominated classes will attempt to limit the power of those in authority over them. Given this, it is now possible to see in these acts of resistance, located as they are at the level of practical activity - production, the link between social action and social consciousness. A link that if viewed critically does not fall prey to voluntarism and subjectivism.

Like Giddens' work, this notion must be predicated on acting and rational subjects and it is here that I wish to turn to the work of Willis and Corrigan (1983). They start their analysis following up their paper of 1980 ("Cultural forms and class mediations") where they commented on the contribution of discourse theory to the study of consciousness and where they criticized the ahistorical nature of such analyses. As they write: "Discourses refer only to themselves and not to an external referent" (Willis and Corrigan, 1983, p86). Therefore it is impossible to choose between one discourse and another. Even more importantly, as we have pointed out before, there is no "reality" which can structure the discourse. All of this is in complete contradiction with what they wish to argue. Moreover, they are concerned with the questions of agency, subjectivity and experience. Likewise, they are interested in placing these in the contexts of the specific locations and structures of capitalism:

> We must see how relations, and particularly class relations, are, yes lived, (and you can see the discourse fever red mark margining the text - this "the immediate humanist relapse") but with a formal attention to how this is formed and accomplished in the recalcitrance of symbolic forms and their internal relationships and their relationship to ideological structuration. And this "Living" involves "understandings," forms of subjectivity, and what certainly participants regard as "experience". "Experience" is a major touchstone for how social relationships - often actually submerging them - are appropriated, and very importantly is also the basis for choice and action which (while partly illusory) actually produces specific material outcomes which help to reproduce the class society in much more complex ways with greater plays of possibilities than any ex post facto idealist theoretical account can contain.
>
> (Willis and Corrigan, 1983, p87)

Although, certain of the ideological forms thrown up by capitalism, such as the fetishism of the commodity; the "fair" wage; equality under the law; representative democracy; etc. deeply structure the possibilities of working class consciousness, it must be still realised that the working class contains resources through which the present set of social arrangements could be radically transformed. This is because they suffer the most collectively and systematically from those social arrangements; "thus subordination makes the working class most open to the determination of capitalist forms and most likely to penetrate resist and overthrow them. Both sides of these possibilities must be kept in play in our specific analysis of concrete "discourses" of culutral forms" (Willis and Corrigan, 1983, p88).

What stems from this argument is that the notion of a dominant ideology, hermetically sealed from contradiction, and being diffused through a variety of media is very much an over pessimistic view. On the contrary, what Willis and Corrigan argue is that the fact that the dominated subjects are able to rationalise the "fit" between the "obvious" and their experience of it, not only means that it is impossible to regard them as "cultural dopes" to use Giddens' phrase, but that it also limits the forms and contents of the ideologies disseminated by the media. Summing up their disagreements with discourse theory they state:

> Class relations form a repertoire of submerged fractured, fissured, contradictory, and semi-visible "resources" from which social individuals, especially through their collective life can simultaneously hold off the dominant social imagery and establish, however partially ways through to a different form of socialisation. We want to argue for a notion of cultural forms as those structured relationships and symbolic systems through which - dialectically together under the impulses of the production of material life - social experiences are formed, felt, framed, sensed, expressed, and transmitted.
> (Willis and Corrigan, 1983, p89)

However, it would be mistaken to believe that in criticising discourse theory from this perspective, the two writers are in fact resurrecting a simple base-superstructure model of working class consciousness where the economic position of the working class forces it to adopt a "true" consciousness of its subjection and, therefore, a clear understanding of what needs to be done. Willis and Corrigan reject this charge of "historicism". "The processes and practices we've discussed cannot bring about any kind of pure expression and are not a direct, one-to-one relation to economic location or to the political possibilities of changing economic structure" (Willis and Corrigan, 1983, p98).

This means that the cultural forms adopted by the working class are not always the ones associated with traditional analyses of class consciousness - the ways in which male working class school culture depreciates mental ability and exalts physical prowess is one example taken from Willis's own classic study "Learning to Labour"(1978). Here the overall result is, as its title suggests, the enabling of capitalism to get the manual labour it needs, while at the same time not to have to deliberately give working class children less of a "chance".

Similarly, this (working class) idea of masculinity also operates in the cultural forms generated in production and is often tied in directly to more conventional forms of class activity:

> In the school and in the factory the whole discourse of masculinity, of masculine presence is often used as a form of opposition to, if you like, class "discourses" of oppression. The exercise of class power through language and cultural 'structured in dominance" (best exposed with references to Marxist categories) is resisted not in straight terms of class consciousness (that one might wish were there) but in what seems to be a discourse which is more controllable by the male working class: masculine sexism and machism.
>
> (Willis and Corrigan, 1983, p92)

Because the cultural forms that result from the contradictions and antagonisms of society are not specifically determined but are created out of the resources to hand Willis and Corrigan argue that some of the stability of capitalism in Britain results from the strengths and richness of working class cultural forms. Again as they write: "the very success of that particularly British form of working class culture can ironically being about its containment" (Willis and Corrigan, 1983, p100).

Turning to the traditional concern of Marxist class analysis, namely the possibility of the development of socialist consciousness their arguments are particularly pertinent:

> We are thus arguing that although there is no sense whatsoever in seeing the cultural forms of resistance as being already available forms of socialist politics, no socialistconstruction is possible that ignores the persistent recurring vibrancy of such resistance. Further, in a highly changeable set of relations (around new technology, for example, let alone the wider crisis of energy and legitimacy,) such forms of resistance can be channeled for right wing proto-fascist chauvinist oppositions, for nostalgic defence of a country, groups or locality. A Marxist dismissal of cultural forms plays into the hands of both the individualising practices of bourgeois hegemony and these fascist (racist, sexist, patriotic) organisations.
>
> (Willis and Corrigan, 1983, p102)

The position outlined above makes more useful Gramsci's notion of dual consciousness. It does so by showing how culture, which is the mediated form of consciousness, is not merely passive but is indeed creative. Obviously, this creativeness is determined by the dominant structures in capitalist society as well as by the balance of class forces. In this way we can solve the problem of agency and structure. However, as Johnson (1979) points out, we must be aware that in seeing the advantages of a culturalist perspectivewe do not to become over-concerned with the description of the cultural processes to the detriment of having a theoretical understanding of the contexts in which they occur, and that consequently we do not reduce the latter into the former. As he writes:

> Any analysis of "working class culture" must be able to grasp the relations between economic classes and the forms in which they do (or do not) become active in conscious politics. If the two aspects of class analysis are conflated this is not possible. If class is only understood as a cultural and political formation, a whole theoretical legacy is impoverished and materialist accounts are indistinguishable from a form of idealism.
>
> (Johnson, 1979, p223)

With this proviso accepted, we have now a theoretical understanding of the consciousness towards privatisation held by the ancillary workers studied earlier. It is capable of understanding the contradictions held by this group by basing them in the practices in which they, as subjects, were involved. This is superior to the analysis offered by discourse theorists because it is grounded at the level of reality. In contradiction to Marxists, discourse theorist and their successors argue that reality, through the medium of economically defined classes, cannot be expressive. Discursive practices are what count; "The "discourse" always expresses or "is" dominance and the dominated have no way "back" into the "discourse" to challenge this position. Dominance is sealed in discursively and the dominated sealed out economically (because of the non-reductiveness of discourse to economic class)" (Corrigan and Willis, 1980, p300).

Discourse theory, therefore, can only accept "the assertion that the working class is totally prone in the face of endlessly repeated subordinate positionings in discourses, texts, and ideology" (Corrigan and Willis,1980, p300).

To conclude it is worth quoting Femia (1975) and his summarising of Gramsci's position. It is worth doing this because within it he describes in essence the conception of ideology that has guided this work:

...despite his lack of familiarity with questionnaires and computers, Gramsci comprehended what appear to be the salient features of mass consciousness in those advanced capitalist societies where Communist Parties have made no inroads. To begin with, he understood that the average individuals belief system is internally contradictory; yet he also recognised the widespread, if somewhat equivocal, acceptance of perceptions and values favorable to the status quo.

...members of subordinate classes come to accept the dominant network of beliefs as an abstract version of reality, but their life conditions weaken its binding force in the actual conduct of affairs.
(Femia, 1975, p46)

Notes

1. Practical consciousness is defined by Giddens as "tacit knowledge that is skillfully applied in the enactment of courses of conduct, but which the actor is not able to formulate discursively"(Giddens,1979, p57), in other words, a practical knowledge of the limits and possibilities of action.

Conclusion

The General Election campaign of 1987 provides a backdrop against which the ideas outlined in this work can be evaluated. It was an election that Labour dominated and many thought won in terms of its campaign. In the end, however, Labour lost and ended up with fewer votes than in 1979 (but with more than in 1983).

The size of the Conservative majority in the House of Commons is not important as this mainly reflects the vagaries of the electoral system. What is of more consequence was the nature of the Labour vote across the country.

Here the geographical spread   reflected a class bias as well as a regional one. Labour did well in traditional working class areas such as Scotland and the North of England; areas that had experienced higher levels of unemployment and industrial decline than other regions. In the South and Midlands its vote changed little or even fell (as it did in London). Though many pointed to this as indicating a North - South divide, what it really pointed to was the different ways in which the recession affected different parts of the country. It was this that created varying electoral swings. After all, the magnitude of the swings towards Labour was not that large. Labour only picked up an extra million votes - which is still less than in 1931 when it recorded its previous "worst" vote.

It is always difficult to make judgements on the basis of election results, what we can say, is that for large numbers of formerly traditional Labour voters (that is pre-1979) in the Midlands and in London the political attraction of Labour was not strong enough to sway them from voting Conservative or switching to the Alliance. The attempt to create the basis for such a swing by ideological means was part of this failure.

Obviously there are complicating factors such as the existence of the Alliance parties and the defence debate, but the fact remains that the issues that Labour campaigned on such as the NHS were not in themselves capable of changing peoples outlooks. It would appear that traditional factors such as jobs and housing were the ones that brought home the bacon in Labours hinterland of support. Whereas outside of these traditional areas Labour did badly (in comparison) because people had jobs and were relatively prosperous. It is a fact that real earnings had increased considerably since 1979.

Labour's strategy of winning an election on the basis of stressing its caring image, and of projecting the NHS as an embodiment of the party simply didn't do the job. In this the central arguments of this work would seem to be vindicated. The whole notion of attempting to change peoples' ideas by waging a counter-hegemonic campaign is one that foundered on its misunderstanding of the nature of peoples' consciousnesses. That these consciousnesses are contradictory and that contradiction is rooted in peoples' practical activities was lost on them. The Labour and Trade Union leaders perceived need for hegemony to be based on TV images and moral invocations rather than on the class struggle also ensured that when opportunities arose (the miners' strike, the News International printworkers' strike, etc.) their full potential was not grasped and the Tories reaped the rewards. More importantly it also meant that the one major strength that the Labour party possesses, its link with the trade unions, was ignored. Many of the areas around London that remained Conservative are not dissimilar to areas further north which deliver majorities to Labour. A significant difference may be the apparent lack of any labour movement traditions or culture. In disavowing industrial militancy the Labour party might have prevented the growth of such traditions and of the support that ensues from it.

The alternative that this work offers is a more practical understanding of consciousness and its capacity for change and for changing the world around it. It emphasises the importance of the practical activities of human subjects in the development of political ideas and movements. It also recognises that these activities may lead to an acceptance of ideas and ideologies that do not represent the best interests of the dominated classes. In addition, the exploitative nature of class divided societies leads continually to those dominated classes coming into conflict with their exploiters and needing to develop ideas and politics to understand these situations.

With an acceptance of the role of the active subject in the maintenance and overcoming of ideological forms, it is possible to construct strategies for social change that have a possibility of success built into them. By concentrating on episodes of class conflict where the potential conflict between exploiting and exploited classes is greatest, it is possible for socialist organisations to develop, among a minority at least, the partial understandings of society that are represented by trade unionism, Labourism, etc. into fuller understandings of the economic basis of capitalism as a system of exploitation. Socialist organisations with an orientation to the class struggle, and by virtue of the minority that agreed with them, would then be able to provide an organic leadership to those struggles which in turn would affect those more subject to the dominant ideologies and move them in a positive direction. This is obviously not a reformist strategy and neither is it one capable of quickly winning peoples' agreement. It attempts to create a socialist hegemony not reflect a bourgeois one.

In this way, the combination of activity and theory can provide a basis for social transformation. Obviously, this begs the question(s) of how precisely to do it, but if it could be achieved, the working class by virtue of its position in society has the power to replace the unequal and alienating social structure it is presently subject to. Why this hasn't occurred as yet, is in some part due to the enticements that other routes to a better world seem to offer. However, like all get rich quick schemes, the promises don't match up to the results, and people seem to find themselves in a worse position than when they started. Maybe one of the positive things to come out of this (continuing) "impasse" of Labourism will be the rediscovery and general acceptance of "left" critiques of social democracy as an alternative to the "right" ones that have had the ascendency for so long.

Bibliography

All references are to works published in London unless otherwise stated.

Abercrombie N. Hill S. and Turner B. (1980) - *The Dominant Ideology Thesis*, Allen and Unwin.

Abercrombie N. (1980) - *Class Structure and Knowledge: Problems in the Sociology of Knowledge*, Basil Blackwell, Oxford.

Adamson W. (1980) - *Hegemony and Revolution: A Study of Antonio Gramsci's Political and Cultural Theory*, California University Press, Berkeley.

Althusser L. (1971) - *Lenin and Philosophy*, Monthly Review Press, New York.

Althusser L. (1979) - *For Marx*, Verso.

Althusser L. and Balibar E. (1979) - *Reading Capital*, Verso.

Altvatar A. (1978) - *Some Problems of State Intervention*, in: Holloway and Picciotto (eds).

Anderson P. (1977) - The Antinomies of Antonio Gramsci, *New Left Review* 100.

Anderson P. (1980) - *Arguments Within English Marxism*, Verso.

Anderson P. (1983) - *In the Tracks of Historical Materialism*, Verso.

Arato A.(1972) - Lukacs' Theory of Reification, *Telos* 11, St Louis, Missouri.

Arato A. and Breines P. (1979) - *The Young Lukacs and the Origins of Western Marxism*, Pluto.

Ascher K. (1987) - *The Politics of Privatisation: Contracting Out Public Services*, St Martin's.

Bacon R. and Eltis W. (1976) - *Britain's Economic Problem: Too Few Producers*, Macmillan.

Barker C. (1978) - The State as Capital, *International Socialism*, series 2. no. 1.

Barrett M. (1980) - *Womens Oppression Today: Problems in Marxist / Feminist Analysis*, Verso.

Barrett Brown M.(1980) - *Models in Political Economy*, Penguin, Harmondsworth.

Bartlett W. (1991) - *Quasi-Markets and Contracts: A Markets Hierarchies Perspective on NHS Reform*, SAUS, Bristol.

Baumol W. (1967) - The Macro-Economics of Unbalanced Growth: the Anatomy of Urban Crisis, *American Economic Review*, 57, 1967.

Beale J. (1983) - *Getting It Together - Women as Trade Unionists*, Pluto.

Beardwell A. (1981) - Low Pay Among Civil Service Cleaners, *Low Pay Review*, no 4.

Benn S. and Gaus G.(eds)(1983) - *Public and Private in Social Life*, Croom Helm, Beckenham.

Bennett T. (1971) - *Formalism and Marxism*, Methuen.

Benton T. (1984) - *The Rise and Fall of Structural Marxism: Althusser and his Influence*, Macmillan.

Birch A.H. (1984) - Overload Ungovernability and Delegitimation: the theories and the British case, *British Journal of Political Science*, vol 14 no 2.

Boddy M. and Fudge C. (1984) - *Labour Councils and New Left Alternatives*, in: Boddy and Fudge (eds), 1984.

Boddy M. and Fudge C. (1984) - *Local Socialism*, Pluto.

Bosanquet N. (1982) - Living with cash limits: the case of the National Health Service, *Public Money*, September, 1982.

Bosanquet N. (1983) - *After the New Right*, Heinneman.

Bosanquet N.(1985) - *Welfare Needs, Welfare Jobs, and Welfare Efficiency*, in Klein and O'Higgins (eds), 1985.

Bosanquet N. (1986) - comment in *Social Expenditure 1960-1990: A Symposium*, .

Brennen G. and Buchanan J.M. (1977) - Towards a tax constitution for Leviathan, *Journal of Public Economics* 9.

Brittan S. (1975) - The Economic Contradictions of Democracy, *British Journal of Political Science*, vol 5 no 1.

Brown D. and Baldwin S.(eds)(1980) - *The Yearbook of Social Policy*,

Routledge and Kegan Paul, 1980.

Buci-Glucksmann C. (1980) - *Gramsci and the State*, Lawrence and Wishart.

Bulmer M. (1975) - *Working Class Images of Society*, Routledge and Kegan Paul, London.

Callinicos A. (1982) - *Is there a future for Marxism?*, Methuen, London.

Callinicos A. (1983) - The New Middle Class and Socialist Politics *International Socialism*, series 2. no 20.

Callinicos A. (1985a) - The Politics of "Marxism Today", *International Socialism*, series 2. no 30.

Callinicos A. (1985b) - *Marxism and Philosophy*, Oxford University Press, Oxford.

Callinicos A. (1985c) - Anthony Giddens - A Contemporary Critique, *Theory and Society*, no 14.

Cameron D. (1985) - *Public Expenditure and Economic Performance in International Perspective*, in: Klein and O'Higgins (eds), 1985.

Cameron D. (1984) - *Social Democracy, Corporatism, Labour Quiescence and the Representation of Economic Interest in Advanced Capitalist Society*, in: Goldthorpe (ed), 1984.

Campbell B. (1984) - *Wigan Pier Revisited*, Virago.

Campbell B. (1985) - Politics Old and New, *New Statesman*, 11th March.

Carlin N. and Birchall I. (1983) - Kinnock's Favorite Marxist: Eric Hobsbawm and the Working Class, *International Socialism*, series 2. no 21.

Carter R. (1985) - *Capitalism, Class Conflict and the New Middle Class*, Routledge and Kegan Paul.

Centre for Contemporary Cultural Studies. (ed) (1977) - *On Ideology*, Working Papers in Cultural Studies no 10, University of Birmingham.

Clarke S. (ed) (1979) - *Working Class Culture*, Hutchison/ Centre for Contemporary Cultural Studies.

Cockburn C. (1977) - *The Local State*, Pluto.

Cockburn C. - *Brothers: Male Dominance and Technological Change*, Pluto, 1983.

Cohen I. (1987) - *Structuration Theory and Social Praxis*, in Giddens and Held (eds), 1987.

Cole K. Cameron J. and Edwards C. (1983) - *Why Economists Disagree: The Political Economy of Economics*, Longmans.

Colletti L. (1975) - *Karl Marx - Early Writings*, Introduction by L. Colletti, Penguin, Harmondsworth.

Communist Party. (1989) - *New Times*, Communist Party of Great Britain.

Corrigan P. and Willis P. (1980) - Cultural Forms and Class Mediations,

Media, Culture and Society, no 2.

Coward R. and Ellis J. (1977) - *Language and Materialism: Developments in Semiology and the Theory of the Subject*, Routledge and Kegan Paul.

Coyle A. (1985) - Going Private: the Implications of Privatisation for Women's Work, *Feminist Review*, no 21.

Crewe I. (1982) - *The Labour Party and the Electorate*, in Kavanagh (ed), 1982.

Cronin J.E. (1984) - *Labour and Society in Britain 1918-79*, Batsford Academic and Educational, 1984.

Crouch C.(1979) - *The Politics of Industrial Relations*, Collins.

CSE State Group. (1979) - *Struggle Over the State:Cuts and Restructuring in Contemporary Britain*, CSE Books.

Curran J. (ed)(1984) - *The Future of the Left*, Polity Press/New Socialist, Cambridge University Press.

Dallymar F. (1982) - *The Theory of Structuration: A Critique*, in: Giddens, 1982b.

Dant T. (1991) - *Knowledge, Ideology and Discourse*, Routledge.

Davies B. - Making a reality of Community Care, *British Journal of Social Work*, vol 18 (Supplement).

Davis G. and Piachaud D. (1983) - *Social Policy and the Economy*, in: Glennerster (ed), 1983.

Davis G. and Piachaud D. (1985) - *Public Expenditure on Social services: The Economic and Political Constraints*, in Klein and O'Higgins (eds), 1985.

Davis H. (1989) - *Beyond Class Images*, Croom Helm.

Delphy C. (1977) - *The Main Enemy,* Womens Resources and Research Centre.

Desai M. (1984) - *Economic Alternatives for Labour 1984-1989*, in: Griffiths (ed), 1984.

DHSS (1983)- *Circular 18 / 1983.*

DHSS (1985) - £19 Million a Year Now Being Saved by Competitive Tendering in the NHS, *Press Release 85/234.*

Donnison D. (1984) - *The Progressive Potential of Privatisation*, in: Le Grand and Robinson (eds), 1984.

Downs A. (1960) - Why the Government Budget is too small in a Democracy, *World Politics* 12.

Draper H. (1975) - *Karl Marx's Theory of Revolution; Volume 1, The State and Bureacracy*, Monthly Review Press, New York.

Dunleavy P. (1979) - The Political Implications of Sectoral Cleavages and the Growth of State Employment, pts I and II, *Political Studies,*vol 28, nos 3-4, 1979.

Eagleton T. (1983) - *Literary Theory*, Basil Blackwell, Oxford.

Ellis R. (1985) - Fiscal Policy: Rhetoric and Reality, *Economic Affairs Supplement*, vol 5, no 3.

Engels F.(1978) - *Ludwig Feuerbach and the End of Classical German Idealism*, Progress Publishers, Moscow.

Femia S. (1975) - Hegemony and Consciousness in the Thought of Antonio Gramsci, *Political Studies*, vol 23, no 1.

Femia S. (1981) - *Gramsci's Political Thought; Hegemony and Consciousness, and the Revolutionary Process*, Clarendon Press, Oxford.

Fine B. and Harris L. (1976) - State Expenditure in Advanced Capitalism: A Critique, *New Left Review* 98, 1976.

Fine B. et al; (1985) - *Class politics: An Answer to its Critics,* Leftover Pamphlets.

Firestone S. (1979) - *The Dialectic of Sex*, Womens Press.

Fitzpatrick R. (1987) - *Political Science and Health Policy,* in Scambler (ed) (1987).

Forsyth G. (1982) - *The semantics of health care policy and the inevitability of regulation*, in McLachan and Maynard (eds), 1982.

Foucault M. (1973) - *The Archaeology of Knowledge*, Tavistock.

Frankel B. (1978) - *Marxian Theories of the State: a Critique of Orthodoxy*, Arena Publications Associates, Monograph Series no 3, Victoria, Australia.

Franklin M. (1986) - *The Decline of Class Voting in Britain: Changes in the Basis of Electoral Choice 1964-1983*, Clarendon Press, Oxford.

Freeman S. and Vandesteeg B. (1981) - What is "Unproductive Labour"?, *International Socialism*, series 2. no 12.

Fryer B. Manson T. Fairclough A. (1978) - Employment and trade unionism in the public services, background notes to the struggle against the cuts, *Capital and Class*, no 4.

George V. and Wilding P. (1976) - *Ideology and Social Welfare*, Routledge and Kegan Paul.

Giddens A. (1979) - *Central Problems in Social Theory: Action, Structure and Contradiction in Social Analysis*, Macmillan.

Giddens A. (1982a) - *A Contemporary Critique of Historical Materialism: Volume One: Power, Property and the State*, Macmillan.

Giddens A. (1982b) - *Profiles and Critiques in Social Theory*, Macmillan.

Giddens A. (1982c) - *Power, the Dialectic of Control and Class Structuration*, in Giddens and McKenzie (eds), 1982.

Giddens A. (1985) - Marx's Correct Views on Everything, *Theory and Society*, no 14.

Giddens A. and McKenzie G. (1982c) - *Social Class and the Division of*

Labour, Cambridge University Press, Cambridge.

Giddens A. and Held D. (1987) - *Social Theory Today,* Polity.

Gillion C. and Hemming R. (1985) - *Social Expenditure in the UK in a Comparative Context,* in Klein and O'HIggins (eds), 1985.

Gillion C. and Hemming R. (1986) - *Comment* in Symposium, 1986.

Glennerster H. (1980) - *Public Spending and the Social Services: the end of an era?* in Brown and Baldwin (eds), 1980.

Glennerster H. (ed) (1983) - *The Future of the Welfare State: Remaking Social Policy,* Heinnemann.

Glyn A. and Sutcliffe B.(1972) - *British Capitalism, Workers and the Profit Squeeze,* Penguin, Harmondsworth.

Golding and Middleton, (1983) - *Images of Welfare: Press and Public Attitudes to Welfare and Poverty,* Martin Robertson, Oxford.

Goldthorpe J.H. - *The End of Convergence: Corporatist and Dualist Tendencies in Modern Welfare Societies,*in: Order and Conflict in Contemporary Capitalism, Goldthorpe (ed), Clarendon Press, Oxford, 1984.

Gorz A. (1982) - *Farewell to the Working Class: An Essay on Post-Industrial Socialism,* Pluto.

Gough I. (1976) - State Expenditure in Advanced Capitalism, *New Left Review,* 92.

Gough I. (1979) - *The Political Economy of the Welfare State,* Macmillan.

Gough I. (1983) - The Crisis of the British Welfare State, *International Journal of Health Services,* vol 13 no 3.

Gough I. (1983a) - *Thatcherism and the Welfare State,* in Jacques and Hall (eds), 1983a.

Gramsci A. (1957) - *The Modern Prince and Other Writings,* Lawrence and Wishart.

Gramsci A. (1971) - *Selections From the Prison Notebooks of Antonio Gramsci,* Hoare and Nowell-Smith (eds), Lawrence and Wishart, 1971.

Green P. (1987) - British Capitalism and the Thatcher Years, *International Socialism,* series 2. no 35.

Grey A. (1984) - Real Resources and Unreal Assumptions: the Case of the NHS, *Public Money,* Dec 1984.

Griffin L. et al.(1983) - On the Economic and Political Determinants of Welfare Spending in the Post-World War Two Era, in *Politics and Society,* no 3.

Griffith J.(ed)(1983) - *Socialism in a Cold Climate,* Unwin.

Habermas J. (1976) - *Legitimation Crisis,* Heinnemann.

Haggar T. (1984) - Cash Planning in the NHS, *Health and Social Services Journal,* October, 4 1984.

Hain P. (1986) - *Political Strikes*, Penguin, Harmondsworth, 1985.

Hall D. (1983) - *The Cuts Machine: The Politics of Public Expenditure*, Pluto.

Hall S. (1983) - *The Great moving Right Show*, in Jacques and Hall (eds), 1983.

Hall S. (1984) - *The Crisis of Labourism*, in Curran (ed), 1984.

Hall S. (1985) - Authoritarian Populism: A Reply, *New Left Review* 151.

Hall S. (1985) - Gramsci and Us,*Marxism Today* June, 1985.

Hall S. (1989) - *The Hard Road to Renewal*, Verso.

Hallas D. (1980) - Trade Unionists and Revolution: A Response to Richard Hyman, *International Socialism,* series 2. no 8.

Halpern S. (1985) - The Billion Pound Efficiency Drive, *Health Service Journal,* 29th January, 1985.

Harland R. (1987) - *Superstructuralism: The Philosophy of Structuralism and Post-structuralism*, Methuen.

Harman C. (1979) - The Crisis of the European Revolutionary Left, *International Socialism,* series 2. no 4.

Harman C. (1980) - Marx's Theory of Crisis and its Critics, *International Socialism,* series 2. no 11.

Harman C. (1982) - State Capitalism, Armaments and the General Form of the Current Crisis, *International Socialism*, series 2. no 16.

Harman C. (1984) - *Gramsci Versus Reformism,* Socialist Workers Party.

Harris N. (1983) - *Of Bread and Guns*, Penguin, Harmondsworth.

Hastings S. and Levie H. (eds)(1983) - *Privatisation?*, Spokesman, Nottingham.

Hayek F. (1973) - *Law, Legislation and Liberty*, in *Rules and Order*, vol 1, Routledge and Kegan Paul.

Heald D. (1983) - *Public Expenditure*, Martin Robertson, Oxford.

Heath A. Jowell R. and Curtice J. (1985) - *How Britain Votes,*Pergamon, Oxford.

Heclo and Wildavsky. (1971) - *The Private Government of Public Money,* Macmillan.

Held D. (ed) (1983) - *States and Societies,* Martin Robertson, Oxford.

Hewitt M. (1983) - Bio-Politics and Social Policy, *Theory, Culture and Society,* vol 2 no1.

Hindess B. (1985) - *Parliamentary Democracy and Socialist Politics*, Routledge.

Hinton J. (1983) - *Labour and Society: A History of the British Labour Movement, 1867-1974*, Wheatsheaf, Brighton.

Hirst P. (1977) - *Economic Classes and Politics*, in Hunt (ed), 1977.

219

Hirst P. (1979) - *On Law and Ideology*, Macmillan.

HMSO (1979) - *The Governments Expenditure Plans 1979-80 to 1981-82*, Cmnd 7746, London.

Hobsbawm E. (1981) - *The Forward March of Labour Halted*, in Jacques and Mulhearn (eds), 1981.

Hogg Q. (1947) - *The Case for Conservatism*, Penguin, Harmondsworth.

Holloway J. and Picciotto S. (eds), (1978) - *State and Capital: a Marxist Debate*, Edward Arnold.

Hook S. (1965) - *From Hegel to Marx; Studies in the Intellectual Development of Karl Marx*, Ann Arbor Press, Michigan.

Hunt A. (ed) (1975) - *Class and Class Structure*, Lawrence and Wishart.

Hyman R. (1971) - *Marxism and the Sociology of Trade Unionism*, Pluto.

Hyman R. (1980) - British Trade Unionism: Post-War Trends and Future Prospects, *International Socialism*, series 2. no 8.

Hyman R. (1984) - *Wooing the Working Class*, in Curran (ed), 1984.

Iliffe S. (1983) - *The NHS - A Picture of Health*, Lawrence and Wishart.

Iliffe S. (1985) - The Politics of Health Care: the NHS under Thatcher, *Critical Social Policy*, no 14.

Jacques M. and Mulhearn F.(1981) - *The Forward March of Labour Halted*, Lawrence and Wishart.

Jacques M. and Hall S. (1983) - *The Politics of Thatcherism*, Lawrence and Wishart.

Jefferys S. (1979) - Striking into the 1980s - Modern British Trade Unionism: its Limit and Potential, *International Socialism*, series 2. no 5.

Jessop B. (1980) - *The Political Indeterminacy of Democracy*, in Hunt (ed), 1980.

Jessop B. (1982) - *The Capitalist State; Marxist Theories and Methods*, Martin Robertson, Oxford.

Jessop B. (1986) - *Nicos Poulantzas: Marxist Theory and Political Strategy*, Macmillan.

Jessop B. et al. (1984) - Authoritarian Populism, Two Nations and Thatcherism, *New Left Review* 147.

Jessop B. et al. (1985) - Thatcherism and the Politics of Hegemony: A Reply to Stuart Hall, *New Left Review* 153.

Johnson P. (1978) - The Promise of Public Sector Unionism, *Monthly Review* vol 30, no4.

Johnson R. (1979) - *Three Problematics: Elements of a Theory of Working Class Culture*, in Clarke (ed), 1979.

Jones C. (1983) - *State Social Work and the Working Class*, Methuen.

Jowell R. and Airey C. (1984) - *British Social Attitudes - The 1984 Report*, Gower, Aldershot.

Jowell R. and Witherspoon S. (1985) - *British Social Attitudes - The 1985 Report*, Gower, Aldershot.

Jowell R. Witherspoon S. and Brook L.(1986) - *British Social Attitudes - The 1986 Report*, Gower, Aldershot.

Judge K. (1982) - *The Growth and Decline of Social Expenditure*, in Walker (ed), 1982.

Judge K. and Knapp M. (1985) - *Efficiency in the Production of Welfare: The Public and Private Sectors Compared*, in Klein and O'Higgins (eds), 1985.

Kitching G. (1983) - *Rethinking Socialism*, Spokesman.

Klein R. (1976) - The Politics of Public Expenditure: American Theory and British Practice, *British Journal of Political Science*, vol 6.

Klein R. (1983) - *The Politics of the National Health Service*, Longmans, Harlow.

Klein R. (1984) - Privatisation and the Welfare State, *Lloyds Bank Review*, January, 1984.

Klein R. and O'Higgins M. (1985) - *The Future of Welfare*, Basil Blackwell, Oxford.

Klein R. and Scrivens E. (1986) - The Welfare State - From Crisis to Uncertainty, in *Symposium*, 1986

Knapp M. - Searching for Efficiency in Long-Term Care: De-institutionalisation and Privatisation, *British Journal of Social Work*, vol 18 (Supplement).

Labour Party (1976) - *Proceedings of 1976 Conference*, Labour Party.

Laclau E. (1979) - *Politics and Ideology in Marxist Theory*, Verso.

Laclau E. and Mouffe C. (1982) - Recasting Marxism: Hegemony and New Political Movements, *Socialist Review* (U.S.), no 66.

Laclau E. and Mouffe C. (1985) - *Hegemony and Socialist Strategy*, Verso.

Laing W. (1982) - Contracting Out in the NHS, in *Public Money*, December, 1982.

Laing and Cruikshank. (1984) - Prospects for Privatisation, *Contract Services*, January/February, 1984.

Larrain J. (1979) - *The Concept of Ideology*, Hutchison.

Larrain J. (1983) - *Marxism and Ideology*, Macmillan.

Lash S. and Urry J. (1987) - The Shape of Things to Come, *New Socialist*, January, 1987.

Laurance J. (1986) - Waiting to Clean Up, *New Society*, 18th July, 1986.

Le Grand J. (1984) - The Future of the Welfare State, *New Society*, June 7th, 1984.

Le Grand J. (1983) - *Privatisation and the Social Services*, in Griffith J.(ed),1983.

Lenin V. (1977) - *The State and Revolution: The Marxist Theory of the State and the Tasks of the Proletariat in the Revolution*, Progress Publishers, Moscow.

Leonard P. (1979) - Restructuring the Welfare State: From Social Democracy to the Radical Right, *Marxism Today*, December, 1979.

Linton M. (1986) - The Born Again Labour Voters,in *New Society*, 26th September,1986.

London Edinburgh Weekend Return Group. (1979) - *In and Against the State, Discussion Notes for Socialists*, LEWERG.

London CSE Group. (1980) - *The Alternative Economic Strategy*, CSE Books.

Lovell T. (1980) - *Picture of Reality: Aesthetics, Politics and Pleasure*, British Film Institute.

Lukacs G. (1971) - *History and Class Consciousness*, Merlin, 1971.

McAllister I. and Mughan A. (1985) - Attitudes, Issues and Labour Party Decline in England 1974 - 79, *Comparative Political Studies*, vol 18 no 1.

McCarney J. (1980) - *The Real World of Ideology*, Harvester, Hassocks.

McDonough R. (1979) - *Lukacs; Ideology as False Consciousness*, in CCCS (ed), 1977.

McLachan D. and Maynard A (eds). (1982) - *The Public/Private Mix for Health: the Relevance and Effects of Change*, Nuffield Provincial Hospitals Trust, 1982.

McLennan G. Molina V. and Peters R. (1977) - *Althusser's Theory of Ideology*, in CCCS (ed), 1977.

Mann M. (1973) - *Consciousness and Action Among the Western Working Class*, Macmillan.

Marshall G. (1983) - Some Remarks on the Study of Working Class Consciousness, in *Politics and Society*, vol 12 no 3, 1983.

Marshall G. Newby H. Rose D. Vogler C. (1988) - *Social Class in Modern Britain*, Hutchison.

Marx K. (1973) - *Grundrisse*, Penguin, Harmondsworth.

Marx K. (1976) - *Capital*, volume 1, Penguin, Harmondsworth.

Marx K. and Engels F. (1975) - *Collected Works*, volume 4, Lawrence and Wishart.

Maynard A. and Ludbrook A. (1980) - Budget Allocation in the National Health Service, *Journal of Social Policy*, vol 9.

Maynard A. and Williams M. (1984) - *Privatisation and the NHS*, in LeGrand and Robinson (eds), 1984.

Middlemas R. (1979) - *Politics in Industrial Society: The Experience of the British System Since 1911*, Andre Deutch.

Miliband R. (1985) - The New Revisionism in Britain, in *New Left Review* 150.

Minford P. (1984) - State Expenditure: A Study in Waste, in *Economic Affairs Supplement*, April/June, 1984.

Mishra R. (1984) - *The Welfare State in Crisis - Social Thought and Social Change*, Wheatsheaf, Brighton.

Mishra R. (1986) - The left and the Welfare State: A Critical Analysis, *Critical Social Policy*, no 15.

Mohan J. (1986) - *Restructuring in the Health Sector: Implications for Health Care Provision and Employment*, Paper presented to ESRC meeting on the Changing Urban and Regional System, 1986.

Mohan J. and Woods K. (1985) - Restructuring Health Care: The Social Geography of Public and Private Health Care Under the British Conservative Government, *International Journal of Health Services*, vol 15 no 2.

Molyneaux J. (1978) - *Marxism and the Party*, Pluto Press.

Moor W. (1987) - Building a Public Health Alliance, *Health Services Journal*, 23rd July, 1987.

Mouffe C. (1983) - Working Class Hegemony and the Struggle for Socialism, in *Studies in Political Economy*, 12.

Mullard M. (1985) - *The Politics of Public Expenditure: A Study of Changes in Public Expenditure in Britain since 1970*, M Phil Thesis, University of Southampton.

Muller W. and Neususs C. (1978) - *The Welfare State Illusion and the Contradiction between Wage Labour and Capital*, in Holloway and Picciotto (eds), 1978

Navarro V. (1978) - *Class Struggle, the State and Medicine: An Historical and Contemporary Analysis of the Medical Sector in Great Britain*, Martin Robertson.

Neale J. (1983) - *Memoirs of a Callous Picket: Working for the NHS*, Pluto.

New Left Review (eds) (1978) - *Western Marxism: A Critical Reader*, Verso.

Niskanen W. (1971) - *Bureaucracy and Representative Government*, Aldine/Atherton, Chicago.

Nozick R. (1974) - *Anarchy, State and Utopia*, Basil Blackwell, Oxford.

O'Connor J. (1973) - *The Fiscal Crisis of the State*, St Martins Press, New York.

O'Connor J. (1981) - The fiscal Crisis of the State Revisited: A Look at Economic Crisis and Reagan's Budget Policy, *Kapitalistate*, no 9.

Offe C. (1984) - *Contradictions of the Modern Welfare State*, Hutchison.

O'Higgins M. (1982) - *Rolling Back the Welfare State*, in Walker (ed), 1982.

O'Higgins M. and Patterson A. (1984) - *The Prospects for Public Expenditure or Modelling Through Out of the Crisis*, Paper to ESRC conference on social policy and the economy:-the future of the welfare state, Bath, June 1984.

Panitch L. (1971) - Ideology and Integration: The Case of the British Labour Party, *Political Studies*, vol 19 no 2.

Panitch L. (1976) - *Social Democracy an Industrial Militancy: The Labour Party, The Trade Unions and Incomes Policy*, Cambridge University Press, Cambridge.

Panitch L. (1980) - Recent Theorisations of Corporatism: Reflections on a Growth Industry, *British Journal of Sociology*, vol 31 no 2, 1980.

Panitch L. (1986) - The Impasse of Social Democratic Politics, in *Socialist Register* 1985/86.

Papadakis E. and Taylor-Gooby P. (1987) - *The Private Provision of Public Welfare*, Wheatsheaf.

Paul J. (1984) - Contracting Out in the NHS: Can We Afford to Take the Risk, *Critical Social Policy*, no 10.

Peacock A. (1984) - Privatisation in Perspective, *Three Banks Review*, no 144.

Pecheaux M. (1982) - *Language, Semantics, and Ideology*, Macmillan.

Pliatzky L. (1982) - *Getting and Spending: Public Expenditure Employment and Inflation*, Basil Blackwell, Oxford.

Pollert A. (1981) - *Girls, Wives, Factory Lives*, Macmillan.

Posner M. (1982) - Privatisation: The Frontier between Public and Private, *Policy Studies*, 5 (1).

Poulantzas N. (1975) - *Classes in Contemporary Capitalism*, New Left Books.

Poulantzas N. (1978) - *Political Power and Social Classes*, Verso.

Poulantzas N. (1980) - *State, Power, Socialism*, Verso.

Public Money (1983) - Pay and Disputes in the NHS, *Public Money*, December, 1983.

Public Money. (1984) - Public Versus Private Provision: What People Think? *Public Money*, December 1984.

Radical Statistics Health Group. (1986) - Unsafe in their Hands, Health Service Statistics for England, *International Journal of Health Services*,vol 16 no 2.

Rawls J. (1971) - *A Theory of Justice*, Clarendon Press, Oxford.

Reid I. and Wormold E. (1982) - *Sex Differences in Britain*, Grant McIntyre.

Robinson R. (1986) - Restructuring the Welfare State: an analysis of

Public Expenditure 1979/80-1984/85, *Journal of Social Policy*, vol 15 no 1.

Roiser M. (1987) - Is there a Public Opinion, *Socialist Worker Review*, no 9.

Sanders D. Ward H. Marsh D. (1987) - Government Popularity and the Falklands War: A Reassessment, *British Journal of Political Science*, vol 17.

Sanders D. (1991) - Government Popularity and the Next General Election, *Political Quarterly*, vol 64.

Saunders P. (1985) - Public Expenditure and Economic Performance in OECD Countries, *Journal of Public Policy*, vol 5 no 1.

de Saussure F. (1966) - *Course in General Linguistics*, Peter Owen.

Schmitter P. (1974) - Still the Century of Corporatism? *Review of Politics* 36.

Seldon A. (1980) - *The Litmus Papers*, Centre for Policy Studies.

Sherman J. (1984) - Trading Places - Domestic Managers and Privatisation, *Health and Social Service Journal*, January 26th, 1984.

Showstack-Sassoon S. (1982) - *Approaches to Gramsci*, Readers and Writers.

Singer P. (1983) - *Hegel*, Oxford University Press, Oxford.

Statham C. (1978) - *Radicals in Social Work*, Routelege and Kegan Paul.

Stedman Jones G. (1978) - *The Marxism of the Early Lukacs*,in New Left Review (eds), 1978.

Stedman Jones G. (1984a) - *Languages of Class: Studies in English Working Class History*, Cambridge University Press, Cambridge.

Stedman Jones G. (1984b) - *Marching into History*, in Curran (ed), 1984,

Sumner C. (1979) - *Reading Ideologies: an Investigation into the Marxist Theory of Ideology and Law*, Academic Press.

Symposium. (1986) - Social expenditure: 1960-1990: Problems of Growth and Control, *Journal of Public Policy*, vol 5 no 2.

Tarschys D. (1986) - Comment in *Symposium*.

Taylor-Gooby P. (1981) - The State, Class Ideology and Social Policy, *Journal of Social Policy*, vol 10 no 2.

Taylor-Gooby P. (1984a) - *The Politics of Welfare: Public Attitudes and Behaviour*, Paper presented to ESRC conference on the "Future of Welfare", Bath, June, 1984.

Taylor-Gooby P. (1984b) - *Pleasing any of the people some of the time: Perceptions of redistribution and attitiudes to welfare*, Paper prepared for Government and Opposition workshop on politics of the welfare state, Manchester, September, 1984.

Taylor-Gooby P. (1985) - *Public Opinion, Ideology and State Welfare*, Routledge and Kegan Paul.

Therborn G. (1980) - *The Power of Ideology and the Ideology of Power*, Verso.

Therborn G.(1984) - The Prospects for Labour and the Transformation of Late Capitalism, *New Left Review* 145.

Thompson E.P. (1978) - *The Poverty of Theory and Other Essays*, Merlin, 1978.

Titmuss R. (1969) - *Commitment to Welfare*, Allen and Unwin.

Tomlinson J. (1985) - *British Macroeconomic Policy since 1940*, Croom Helm, Beckenham.

Tomlinson J. (1986) - *Monetarism: Is There an Alternative Non-Monetarist Strategy for the Economy?*, Basil Blackwell, Oxford.

Travis A. (1987) - Nurses Give Teachers a Lesson, in *Health Services Journal*, 28th May, 1987.

Walker A.(ed) (1982) - *Public Expenditure and Social Policy*, Heinemann.

Walker A. (1982) - *The Political Economy of Privatisation*, in LeGrand and Robinson (eds), 1982

Walton A.S. (1983) - *Public and Private Interests: Hegel on Civil Society and the State*, in Benn and Gauss (eds), 1983.

Weale A. (1986) - Ideology and Welfare, *The Quarterly Journal of Social Affairs*, vol 2 no 3.

Weatherly P. (1988) - Class Struggle and the Welfare State: Some theoretical Problems Considered, *Critical Social Policy*, vol 22.

Weir A. and Wilson E. (1984) - Feminism and Class Politics: The British Womens Movement, *New Left Review*, 148.

Westergaard J.H. (1984) - *The Once and Future Class*,in Curran (ed), 1984.

Whitfield D. (1983) - *Making it Public: Evidence and Action against Privatisation*, Pluto Press.

Whiting H. (1984) - Waiting to Clean Up / Privatisation, in *Health and Social Services Journal*, January 26th, 1984.

Willis P. (1978) - *Learning to Labour*, Saxon House, Farnborough.

Willis P. and Corrigan P. (1983) - Orders of Experience: The Differences of Working Class Cultural Forms. *Social Text* 7.

Wilson E. (1980) - Marxism and the Welfare State (Review of Gough's "Political Economy of the Welfare State"), *New Left Review*, 122.

Wood E.M. (1986) - *The Retreat From Class: A New True Socialism*, Verso.

Wright E.O. (1978) - *Class, Crisis and the State*, New Left Books.

Wright E.O. (1983) - Giddens' Critique of Marxism, *Politics and Society*, vol 12 no 3.

Wright E.O. (1985) - *Classes*, Verso.

Yarrow G. (1986) - Privatisation in Theory and Practice, *Economic Policy*, vol 1 no 2.

Young K. (1985) - *Shades of Opinion,* in: British Social Attitudes Survey, SCPR, Gower, 1985.